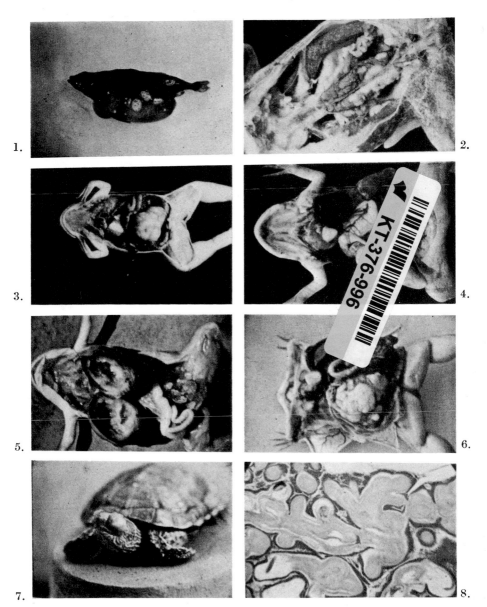

FRONTISPIECE

1. *Gasterosteus aculeatus* infected with *Glugea anomala* and *Schistocephalus solidus*. 2. *Xenopus laevis*. Tuberculosis of kidneys. 3. *Xenopus laevis*. Tuberculosis of rectum. 4. *Xenopus laevis*. Lobar tuberculous pneumonia. 5. *Xenopus laevis*. Biliary adenoma with extensive central necrosis. 6. *Xenopus laevis*. Nephroblastoma. 7. *Clemmys leprosa*. Hyperplasia of Harderian gland. 8. *Chinemys reevesii*. Hyperplasia of Harderian gland. Microscopic section.

PUBLISHER'S PREFACE

The Academic Press (London and New York) published a translation of Dr. Heinz H. Reichenbach-Klinke's *Krankheiten der Aquarienfische* (Diseases of Aquarium Fishes), *Krankheiten der Amphibien* (Diseases of Amphibians) and *Krankheiten der Reptilien* (Diseases of Reptiles). This translation was accomplished by Dr. E. Elkan who is himself an outstanding pathologist.

Published in 1965, the three Reichenbach-Klinke books were issued as a single volume under the title **"The Principal Diseases of Lower Vertebrates."** Dr. Elkan, while making the translation, supplied additional material.

Since its original publication, this volume has been well received and references to it have appeared in many scientific and hobbyist works. It soon was out of print, and T.F.H. undertook the re-publication, breaking the book apart into its original three volumes. People interested in the diseases of snakes might hardly be interested in the diseases of gouramis!

In order to make the book more useful, the complete table of contents and index to the three volumes will be included in each volume. This will enable easy reference to material which might be of interest to workers in overlapping disciplines of ichthyological and herpetological pathologies.

Since Dr. Reichenbach-Klinke has written two new books dealing with fish diseases for T.F.H. Publications and since there are so many references to the original volumes, there are no changes in this reprint from the original volume and the page numbers from the original volume have been preserved with the exception of the index which will appear without folio numbers in the first two volumes.

A complete catalogue of T.F.H. books is available by writing to the publisher.

THE PRINCIPAL DISEASES OF LOWER VERTEBRATES
Book III DISEASES OF REPTILES

H. Reichenbach-Klinke
Technische Hochschule and Bayerische Biologische Versuchsanstalt
Munich, Germany

and

E. Elkan
Group IX Laboratories, Shrodells Hospital, Watford
Hertfordshire, England

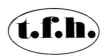

Preface

The "Principal Diseases of Lower Vertebrates" presents the material published by Heinz H. Reichenbach-Klinke between 1957 and 1962 in three separate volumes as "Krankheiten der Aquarienfische" (Alfred Kernen, Stuttgart), "Krankheiten der Amphibien" and "Krankheiten der Reptilien" (Gustav Fischer, Stuttgart). The scope of the work has been enlarged with material contributed by E. Elkan who has also done the translation. We have tried to extend the pathology of fish beyond that of the species kept in aquaria. The scope of fish pathology is, however, widening so rapidly at the present time that no textbook can ever hope to be completely up-to-date even for a short period. Representatives of the main groups of parasites affecting fish have been presented as far as possible.

Experience has shown that those who keep, or are interested in, one kind of lower vertebrate will sooner or later also take an interest in one of the other groups. It was therefore thought expedient to include what is at present known of lower vertebrate pathology in one volume, even at the risk of some repetition where fishes, amphibians and reptiles suffer from similar diseases or are the victims of identical parasites.

Since with the exception, perhaps, of the fishes, the lower vertebrates are of little economic importance, little attention had been paid to their diseases until the day when their usefulness in the laboratory was recognized. Since then, a host of highly technical papers on the pathology and the parasitology of lower vertebrates has appeared in journals inaccessible to the general public. Even so, the textbooks on pathology, bacteriology, zoology and parasitology devote at best only very little space to the diseases of animals not classified as "domestic" or "agricultural".

In trying to fill this gap we have been aware·of the fact that we are dealing with an almost unexplored area of science, and that our knowledge in this field is expanding rapidly. Even so it is hoped that the book may be of use to those interested in any specific problem and may help them to locate the original papers dealing with that particular item.

No attempt has been made to make this book in the widest sense of the word "popular". The disciplines of anatomy, physiology, pathology and zoology are too complicated in their demands of some basic knowledge of the relevant terminology to make that possible. Yet it is hoped that the book—and particularly the illustrations—may be of use to those who keep lower vertebrates for scientific and non-scientific purposes.

If, in many of its parts, this book reads like a pure textbook of parasitology, this is simply due to the fact that, as we descend the evolutionary ladder, more and more diseases are due to parasites and the primary and secondary damage they cause. A basic knowledge of parasitology is therefore indispensable for anyone wanting to keep fish, amphibians or reptiles in good condition.

The production of this book would have been impossible without the kind permission of editors of various scientific journals to reproduce material and illustrations first published in their pages. This refers particularly to the Zoological Society of London, The British Herpetological Society, *Nature*, the *Journal of Protozoology*, *Cancer Research*, *Copeia* and others. To all of them and the many individual authors who gave us permission to use some of their material, we are sincerely grateful.

Acknowledgements are equally due to the German publishers Alfred Kernen Verlag, Stuttgart, and Gustav Fischer Verlag, Stuttgart, who generously allowed us to reproduce material published by them under the titles quoted above and who were kind enough to agree to our plans for this English edition in one volume. Finally we wish to thank Academic Press, London, for their helpful collaboration in the production of this book.

Particular thanks are due to a number of authors who allowed us to use or to photograph some of their material; in particular Dr. E. Amlacher, Berlin, Mr. C. Arme, Leeds, Dr. W. Foersch, Munich, Dr. P. Ghittino, Turin, Dr. W. Meyburg, Bremen, Dr. T. Roskam, Ijmuiden, and also the Bavarian Institute for Experimental Biology, Munich, as well as to two technical assistants in the Department of Chemistry of the same Institute, Miss H. Amtmann and Mr. W. Schlagbauer, who assisted in the execution of some of the drawings.

Since both authors hope to continue working in the field of lower vertebrate pathology they will be grateful to receive relevant material dead or alive. A great deal of collaboration between zoologists, parasitologists and pathologists will be needed before a complete text of lower vertebrate disease can be written.

H. REICHENBACH-KLINKE

January 1965   E. ELKAN

Contents

PART II. AMPHIBIA

PART III. REPTILIA

Part III

Reptilia

CHAPTER 19

Technique of Investigation

A. SYMPTOMS OF DISEASE. AGES OF REPTILES

Like other animals reptiles have to be closely watched if their state of health is to be accurately assessed. Concealment, away from the other inhabitants of the cage, abnormal sluggishness or restlessness may be indications of a bad state of health. Attention should also be paid to difficulties and irregularities in skin shedding and to a loss of the brilliance of the natural colours. Simple measures may sometimes be sufficient to restore the environmental conditions under which the animals have to live to their optimum. The food may be changed or supplemented, the soil improved, the humidity adjusted, sources of light and heat revised. Detailed suggestions concerning these factors will be made in Chapter 26.

One of the most important items in an attempt to diagnose the disease of any animal is a knowledge of its age since advanced age may in itself be responsible for symptoms which, for obvious reasons, cannot be cured. The maximal age attainable by a reptile varies considerably according to the species. Small types like chameleons and lizards are short-lived. Hesse and Doflein (1935) give the following figures:

Species	Years
Scincus officinalis L.	$9\frac{1}{2}$
Uromastix acanthinurus Bell	$9\frac{1}{2}$
Anguis fragilis L.	33

Krefft (1949) gives the following figures for tortoises:

Amyda ferox Schn.	25
Kinosternon subrubrum Lac.	38
Clemmys guttata Tr.	42
Macrochelys temmincki Tr.	42
Terrapene carolina L.	over 100

A Mauritian giant tortoise is said to have lived for 150 years, but the figure of 300 years claimed by Hesse for *Testudo gigantea daudini* D. and B. is of doubtful validity.

The life span of *Testudo graeca* L., one of the reptiles most commonly found in captivity, would interest us particularly. Flower (1944) kept a specimen for 39 years. This tortoise continued to grow to the very end of its life, reached a length of 36·5 cm and a weight of 4 kg. Authors even report on specimens of 54 years of age.

The life span of crocodiles can only be determined in specimens kept in zoological gardens and the figures so obtained are certainly not maximal ones. The greatest, well-authenticated age of a crocodile is 40 years. Brehm ("Tierleben") reports that Nile crocodiles reach the age of "several human generations", also that the natives estimate the age of a crocodile of 5–6 m at about 100 years. None of these estimates are reliable.

Of much greater interest is a report by Dawbin (1962) on the age of the tuatara (*Sphenodon punctatus* Gray). These large lizards grow very slowly and reach sexual maturity only after about 20 years. The author estimates the life span of this species as of 100 years or more.

B. ANAESTHESIA, KILLING OF SPECIMENS, DISSECTION

The removal of external parasites, the painting of ulcerations or other minor items of treatment can, in small animals, be carried out without anaesthesia. It is advisable to envelop the animal with a cloth, leaving only the field of operation exposed. Tails of lizards have to be treated with great respect. Even if a new stump grows after a tail has been cast off, the animal will never be a show specimen again. Larger reptiles can inflict painful and even dangerous bites. Such specimens can only be treated under carefully administered general anaesthesia. The rules governing this procedure are the same as elsewhere, only the dosage must be appropriately reduced. Ether, which is most generally available, can be used on cotton wool in a closed glass jar, but if the animal is not to be killed it must be removed from the jar the very moment it becomes unconscious. "Nembutal" (pentobarbitone sodium, Abbott) can be given by intramuscular or intraperitoneal injection. The dose has to be adjusted according to the weight of the "patient". Urethane, popular in 2–4% solutions for the anaesthesia of aquatic animals, has a depressing effect on the bone-marrow and is now often superseded by M.S. 222 Sandoz, introduced for the anaesthesia of amphibians and fish. It has, apparently, not yet been used on reptilians but these too might lend themselves to the method, used on fish, of

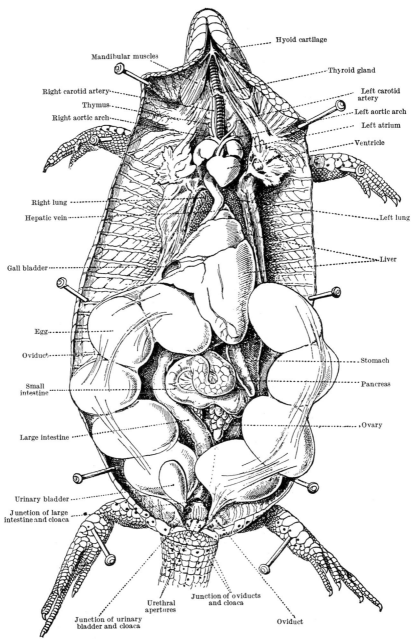

Hyoid cartilage

Mandibular muscles

Thyroid gland

Right carotid artery

Left carotid artery

Thymus

Right aortic arch

Left aortic arch

Left atrium

Ventricle

Right lung

Left lung

Hepatic vein

Gall bladder

Liver

Egg

Oviduct

Stomach

Small intestine

Pancreas

Large intestine

Ovary

Urinary bladder

Junction of large intestine and cloaca

Junction of oviducts and cloaca

Urethral apertures

Junction of urinary bladder and cloaca

Oviduct

FIG. 288. Dissection of a female wall lizard (*Lacerta muralis* L.). (From Kükenthal-Matthes.)

placing a wad of cotton wool, soaked in the solution, into their mouths.

All these chemicals, including chloroform, can in higher doses be used to kill animals too ill to be treated. In addition, the preparations Euthanal (3 cm³ to be injected into the thorax of a medium-sized tortoise) and Nicotin (a small sponge, soaked in the solution, is placed into the animal's mouth) can be used. In particular cases where no drugs are available it may be necessary to decapitate in the region immediately behind the head.

The dissection of all reptilians with the exception of turtles and tortoises can begin with the opening of the visceral cavity from the anus to the thorax. The opening of the peritoneal cavity is particularly important when animals cannot be examined on the spot but have to be fixed and preserved to be sent away to a laboratory. To maintain the integrity of the animal fixation by injection is, of course, preferable, but even a syringe may not always be available. The later dissection of formaldehyde-hardened specimens is much more time-consuming than that of fresh material, but such dissections are made much easier if the specimen has been pinned down fully stretched during fixation.

The skin of reptilians adheres to the superficial fascia and cannot be stripped off without careful use of a very sharp scalpel. On the head, in particular, it is so strongly attached to the bone that a separation is often impossible.

Tortoises can only be dissected after the bridges between the dorsal and ventral shields have been cut either with a wire saw or very strong scissors. Even when this has been done the ventral shield can only be removed after it has been carefully dissected off the underlying muscles.

Bacteriological examination of body fluids is of value in freshly killed specimens only. Blood smears, smears from any other organ and samples of peritoneal fluid should be taken as a first step in the dissection and before any secondary contamination has taken place.

C.   Detailed Examination of Organic Systems

The examination of the various organic systems begins with that of the skin. The axillary and the inguinal folds should be inspected; they are frequently the seat of ticks. Swabs can be taken from ulcers; fresh or stained preparations from exudations may be examined with the aid of the microscope. Cysts or tumours of doubtful nature are either removed *in toto* or fixed together with the surrounding skin so that, in the final section, the relation of the tumour and the skin is maintained.

In the laboratory fixation fluids are chosen according to the staining methods to be employed. Outside the laboratory only alcohol (70%) or formaldehyde (10%) are likely to be available. In either case the specimen should be fixed in at least 10 times its volume of fixing fluid. Further details may be found in textbooks on histological technique.

Muscular and connective tissue are carefully teased in a drop of saline on the microscopic slide and inspected under a cover glass. The digestive tract attracts our attention more than any other organic system since it is most frequently the seat of symbionts and parasites likely to cause disease and death. The oral cavity too should be inspected for parasites, inflammation and ulcers. The intestinal canal should be split along its whole length. In the case of small animals this should be done under saline so that any escaping parasite is not lost but immediately noticed.

Unless it is desired to examine fresh preparations of the bile or the mucous surface of the gall bladder the latter is dissected out together with a portion of the surrounding liver. Both liver and gall bladder are frequently the seat of parasites which can only be detected microscopically.

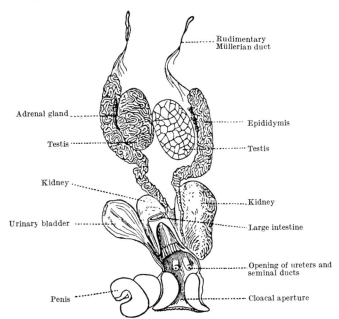

FIG. 289. Urogenital organs of a male wall lizard (*Lacerta muralis* L.). (From Kükenthal Matthes.)

Kidney, ureter, urinary bladder and the gonads should either be examined fresh or in sections. The lungs too are frequently invaded by parasites and bacteria.

Blood smears serve for the detection of parasites and for counts of normal and abnormal cells. Schulz and Krueger (1925) have published the following figures as representing the normal for a few reptilian species:

Species	Erythrocytes	Leucocytes
Emys orbicularis L.	500 000	8 000
Testudo graeca L.	629 000	13 200
Tarentola mauretanica L.	690 000	30 000
Lacerta viridis L.	840 000	
Natrix natrix L.	850 000	8 400
Lacerta agilis L.	0·95–1·29 million	10 500–19 000
Lacerta muralis L.	1–1·6 million	2 000–8 000
Anguis fragilis L.	1·5 million	7 000

On the whole the number of erythrocytes in reptiles varies between 500 000 and 1·5 million mm³; it therefore surpasses that of the Amphibia but does not reach the level of the Mammalia. Figure 290 gives some information on the size of the red blood corpuscles.

Wintrobe (1933) gives the following erythrocyte figures from some reptiles:

Alligator mississippiensis	670 000
Cistudo carolina (Tortoise)	740 000
Freshwater terrapin	740 000
Heterodon contortrix (Snake)	500 000
Heterodon contortrix (Snake)	630 000
Eutaria sirtalis (Garter snake)	1 390 000
Garter snake	710 000
Natrix sipedon (Water snake)	770 000

to which Ryerson (1949) added:

Coleonyx variegatus (Gecko)	491 000
Heloderma suspectum (Gila monster)	646 000
Phrynosoma solare (Horned toad)	745 000
Sceloporus magister (Lizard)	1 224 000
Pituophis sayi (Snake)	1 095 000

Finally Pienaar (1962) gives the following detailed figures for the S. African lizard *Cordylus vittifer*:

Total red count: 790 000–650 000 mm^3 Average 830 000/mm^3
Haemoglobin: 8·0–8·75 g per 100 cc
Length of erythrocytes: 12–18 μ; average 16·5 μ
Width of erythrocytes: 7–10 μ; average 8·5 μ

Parasitic infections as well as seasonal and dietary changes produce severe fluctuations of these figures.

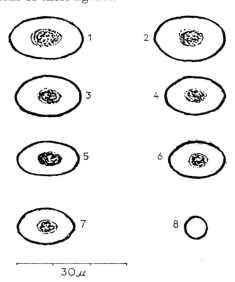

30μ

Fig. 290. Comparison of reptilian and human red blood corpuscles. 1. *Testudo graeca* L. 2. *Emys orbicularis* L. 3. *Natrix natrix* L. 4. *Natrix flavescens* Werner. 5. *Anguis fragilis* L. 6. *Tarentola mauretanica* L. 7. *Lacerta agilis* L. 8. *Homo sapiens* L. (1, 4–7, after Schulz and von Krüger. 2 and 3, after Jung.)

Bernstein (1938) found in *Testudo geometrica* (Tortoise) 642 000 mm^3 and the following four species were examined by Alder and Huber in 1923:

	Erythrocytes
Lacerta agilis	945 000
Anguis fragilis (Slow-worm)	1 615 000
Tarentola mauretanica (Gecko)	692 000
Emys orbicularis (Terrapin)	503 000

To these Pienaar (1962) added:

Agama atra (Lizard)	1 250 000
Chamaeleo dilepis	1 180 000
Cordylus giganteus (Lizard)	650 000

The latest data about other blood constituents of *Cordylus* come from Pienaar (1962):

Leucocytes: Normal variation between 20 000 and 27 000
Thrombocytes: Normal variation from 10 000 to 19 000

Differential normal blood counts of the lizard *Cordylus vittifer* (Pienaar, 1962):

Type of leucocyte	Young ♂♂	Adult ♂♂	Adult ♀♀
Type I eosinophils with spindle-shaped or crystalloid granules	8·64	15·4	13·6
Type II eosinophils with coarse, spheroid granules	0·12	0·18	0·07
Basophil granular lymphocytes (mast myelocytes)	1·00	0·97	0·9
Eosinophil (Type I) myelocytes and metamyelocytes	0·21	1·0	0·33
Basophil (mast) leucocytes	6·38	6·31	6·0
Giant vacuolated "athrocytic" azurophil leucocytes	2·08	0·91	0·8
Typical azurophil granulocytes	1·18	0·54	0·4
Lymphocytoid and plasmacytoid azurophils	3·32	6·8	3·7
Monocytoid azurophils and paramonocytes	0·73	1·35	0·73
Mononuclear neutrophil granulocytes	1·26	2·22	6·2
Large lymphocytes	4·38	4·85	4·57
Medium-sized lymphocytes	20·12	16·83	18·4
Small lymphocytes	48·52	40·01	42·6
Lymphocyte-erythroblast transitions	0·68	0·98	0·44
"Stem-cell" types	1·28	1·65	1·26
Thrombocytes per 100 leucocytes	43·0	48·0	59·0
Erythroblasts and basophilic normoblasts per 100 leucocytes	4·0	6·0	4·0
Polychromasic normoblasts and proerythrocytes per 100 leucocytes	90·0	103·0	53·0
"Megalocytes"—per 100 leucocytes	2·0	4·0	4·0
Mitosing erythrocytes per 500 leucocytes	0–1·0	0–1·0	0–1·0
Binucleate or amitosing erythrocytes per 500 leucocytes	1·0	1–2	1–3
Erythroplastids—per 500 leucocytes	1·0	1·0	1·0

In conformity with repeated observations made by other authors on other vertebrates Pienaar found that it is the eosinophil granulocytes which react most markedly to any abnormal condition. In helminth infections a rise of up to 27% occurred. Eosinophilia was similarly marked in haemoprotozoal infections. In the disease of the Harderian gland of terrapins we can see how large abscesses may even be formed exclusively by eosinophile leucocytes in complete absence of the neutrophile granulocytes usually active in abscess formation. Going by results the neutrophile leucocytes seem to effect a better defence since they produce liquid pus and allow the abscess to break through to the surface and to evacuate itself. The eosinophile leucocytes, however numerous they may be in these glandular abscesses, are unable to do this even if they may sterilize the seat of the original infection. They can therefore never be instrumental to effect a complete cure (p. 518 f.).

Tables of differential blood counts of 23 further S. African reptiles may be found in Pienaar (loc. cit.).

REFERENCES

Cater, D. B. (1953). "Basic Pathology and Morbid Histology." Wright, Bristol.

Dawbin, W. H. (1962). The Tuatara in its natural habitat. *Endeavour* **21**, 16-24.

Flower, S. S. (1944). Persistent growth in the tortoise *Testudo graeca* for thirty-nine years, with other notes concerning that species. *Proc. zool. Soc. Lond.* **114**, 451–455.

Graham-Jones, O. (1961). Notes on the common tortoise. *Vet. Rec.* **73**, 313–323.

Guyer, M. F. (1953). "Animal Micrology." University of Chicago Press.

Hesse, R. and Doflein, F. (1935). "Tierbau und Tierleben", 2nd edn., Fischer, Jena.

Humason, G. L. (1962). "Animal Tissue Techniques." W. H. Freeman. San Francisco.

Jung, T. (1955). Zur Kenntniss der Ernährungsbiologie der in dem Raum zwischen Harz und Heide vorkommenden Hirudineen. *Zool. Jahrb. Phys.* **66**, 79–129.

Klingelhoeffer, W. (1959). "Terrarienkunde." A. Kernen, Stuttgart.

Korschelt, E. (1924). "Lebensdauer, Altern und Tod", 3rd edn., Fischer, Jena.

Krefft, G. (1949). "Die Schildkröten." Wenzel, Braunschweig.

Pienaar, U. de v. (1962). "Haematology of some South African Reptiles." Witwatersrand University Press, Johannesburg, S. Africa.

Romeis, G. (1948). "Mikroskopische Technik." 15th edn., Leibniz, Munich.

Ryerson, D. L. (1949). A preliminary survey of reptilian blood. *J. Ent. Zool.* **41**, 49.

Sandoz A.G. (1961). MS–222. The preferred anaesthetic. *Information Bulletin.*

Schulz, P. N. and v. Krueger, (1925). Das Blut der Wirbeltiere. *In* "Handbuch der vergleichenden Physiologie" (Winterstein, H., ed.), Vol. I. 1. Fischer, Jena.

Smith, H. M. (1957). A record of longevity for the greater five-lined skink. *Herpet.* **13**, 24.

United States Navy (1960). "Manual of Histologic and Special Staining Techniques." The Blakiston Division, McGraw-Hill Book Co.

Wintrobe, M. M. (1933). Variations in size and haemoglobin concentration in the blood of various vertebrates. *Fol. haematol. Lpz.* **51**, 32.

CHAPTER 20

Infectious Diseases

A. BACTERIAL INFECTIONS

Bacterial epizootics are not of unusual occurrence in reptiles. They mainly appear in animals already weakened by other causes and the observations available have mostly been made on caged specimens. The causative bacteria can be divided into two groups according to whether they are themselves the cause of the disease or whether they are merely found on or in the reptile which acts as a carrier. The *Salmonella* group of bacteria often comes into this second category.

Bergey's "Manual of Determinative Bacteriology" (1957) lists the following bacteria as occurring commonly in reptiles:

Pseudomonadales
Enterobacteria
Mycobacteria
Bartonella
Spirochaetales

Pseudomonas reptilivorus was described by Caldwell and Ryerson (1940) from the Mexican beaded lizard *Heloderma suspectum* Cope, from chuckawalla lizards (*Sauromalus ater*) and from the horned toad *Phrynosoma solare* Gray. The strains were described as being equally pathogenic for reptiles, guinea-pigs and rabbits. On autopsy, the animals showed haemorrhagic areas in the stomach, lungs and at the injection site, whilst the liver had assumed a greyish colour. Pseudomonads were recovered by cultivation from heart blood and from peritoneal fluid. They gave rise to marked haemolysis on rabbit blood agar. The authors assumed that an analogous disease occurred among free-living animals.

Pseudomonas fluorescens and *Ps. fl. liquefaciens* are commonly seen in reptiles. The latter was described by Burtscher (1931) as being the causative agent of an ulcerative inflammation of the oral cavity in snakes going by the name of "Mouth Rot". The organism was isolated from fourteen species of snakes including both venomous and non-venomous species. Reinhardt (1927) recorded the same disease as occurring among snakes and lizards kept in zoological gardens. It starts with oedema and inflammation of the oral mucous membrane which swell so much that the animals can no longer close the mouth and are unable to feed (Fig. 291).

Graham Jones (1961) suggests that various fungi supervene and take

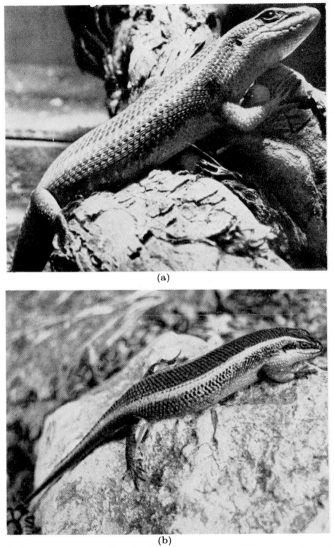

(a)

(b)

FIG. 291. Oral scurvy of reptiles. (a) A skink, *Mabuya striata* Peters. Healthy specimen. (Photo.: Stemmler-Gyger.) (b) The same, suffering from oral scurvy. (Photo.: O. Stemmler-Gyger.)

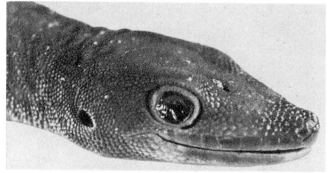

(c)

FIG. 291. (c) A day gecko, *Phelsuma madagascariensis kochi* Mertens which died of oral scurvy. (Orig.)

part in the development of the condition. The idea that ulcerative stomatitis may be caused by more than one agent seems to derive support from occasional successes with vitamin treatment. (O. Stemmler, Basle, personal communication.)

Pseudomonas jaegeri, Ps. smaragdina, Ps. viscosa and *Ps. puris* were isolated by Patrick and Werkman (1930) from a condition in snakes resembling typhoid. A detailed account of the bacteriology and pathology of these species is not yet available.

The same applies to another bacillus, *Pasteurella haemolytica* Newson and Cross, also found in cases of ulcerative stomatitis in reptile collections.

One of the commonest bacteria, always threatening reptile collections, is *Aeromonas hydrophila* (formerly *Proteus hydrophilus*) Sanarelli. This is the bacillus which causes the dreaded disease of "Red Leg" in frogs. Camin (1948) found these bacilli in the heart and in other viscera of snakes. Brison, Tysset and Vacher (1959) found *Testudo graeca* resistant to *Aeromonas* while the aquatic species *Emys orbicularis* was very susceptible.

Equally susceptible is the common grass snake *Natrix natrix* L. as confirmed by the work of Brisou, Tysset and Vacher (quoted by de Rautlin de la Roy, 1960). The authors isolated the bacterium from pus present in the peritoneal cavity as well as from heart blood of grass snakes. *Proteus vulgaris* was isolated from the same material.

Aeromonas can be transmitted by the mite *Ophionyssus serpentinum* Hirst. While the disease could not be directly transmitted from snake to snake, transmission via the mite succeeded in every experiment. Hirst reported mites to be infectious from 48 hours onwards after ingestion of pathogenic bacteria.

The family Enterobacteriaceae (Order Eubacteriales) contains a parasite *Serratia anolium* isolated from the lizard *Anolis equestris* Merr. Clausen and Duran-Reynals (1937) isolated this bacillus from a kind of tumour first from Cuban lizards, later from Mexican iguanids (*Basiliscus vittatus*). They showed the organism to be haemolytic and pathogenic to a wide variety of poikilothermic animals, among them *Anolis equestris*, *A. carolinensis*, *Tarentola mauretanica*, *Hemidactylus brookii*, *Thamnophis butleri*, *Storeria dekayi* and *Sternothaerus odoratus*. They considered the disease as contagious but not necessarily fatal.

The position of "pneumococci", found by Graham-Jones in the lungs of tortoises seems to be systematically uncertain. The bacillus may have been of the genus *Peptostreptococcus*.

Equal uncertainty prevails regarding the description of a *Bacterium sauromali*, Conti and Crowley 1939, found in a specimen of *Sauromalus varius* Dickerson, the "Chuckawalla" of California. The bacillus again caused a kind of tumour in the lizards. The tumours were enclosed in a fibrous capsule and connected with the surrounding tissue by a fibro-vascular neck. The capsule, heavily infiltrated by monocytes, also contained desquamated cells embedded in layers of an amyloid, substance. The tumours were found in the buccal cavity, at the base of the tongue, in the inferior cervical region and in the leg. The bacillus is described as Gram negative, chromogenous, motile but not sporogenous. Full details of the histopathological findings, together with excellent photographs of the condition, are given in the original paper.

The occurrence of the genus *Salmonella* in reptiles is of the greatest importance. Jaksztien and Petzold (1959) reported on *Salmonella* infections of snakes. They were able to identify the serotypes "Arizona", "Charrau", and "Oranienburg" in *Agkistrodon piscivorus* Lacépède, the Water Mocassin snake. One of the snakes dissected was found afflicted with peritonitis, gastric and intestinal inflammation, liver oedema and renal degeneration. Snakes in the early stages of the disease could be cured by intraoral infusion of an aqueous solution of Chloronitrin in doses of 25 cc.

Boycott, Taylor and Douglas (1953) published an extensive report on the occurrence of *Salmonella* in tortoises. Infected specimens seem to be able to carry the most varied serotypes without falling ill themselves. Seventeen such serotypes have so far been recognized, among them "Coruvallis" and "Canastel". Some of these serotypes were found to play a part in human pathology as well. An outbreak of *Salmonella* dysentery in a group of children was thought to have been caused by infected tortoises. Considering the great number of tortoises imported as pets every year the danger does not seem negligible. (See also Buxton (1957) and Kiesewetter *et al.* (1960).)

The occurrence of tuberculosis in reptiles was reviewed by Griffith in 1930. Bergey's manual only mentions *Mycobacterium thamnopheos* Aronson from snakes. *M. tropidonotus* has been reported from *Boa constrictor*, *Coluber catenifer* and *Python molurus*. The names of *M. testudinis* Friedman and Piorkowski and *M. friedmanni* Holland (= *M. cheloni* Bergey *et al.*) are no longer considered valid. The many cases of cold-water tuberculosis seen in reptiles are, on the other hand, doubtlessly not all due to *M. thamnopheos*. Griffith (loc. cit.) separates types pathogenic for turtles (Friedmann's turtle strain), a snake strain and several crocodile strains, among them one for the cayman. The clinical picture is that of typical tuberculosis with pulmonary tubercles (tortoises, turtles) and analogous lesions in skin, liver and spleen (snakes and crocodiles).

Spirochaeta have on several occasions been found both in snakes and in lizards but it is very doubtful whether they should be regarded as pathogenic for these hosts. It is equally uncertain whether the spirochaetes found belong to the genus *Spirochaeta* or *Treponema*. Both names have been used: *Treponema* for lizards; *Spirochaeta* for snakes (Breed, Murray and Hitchens, 1957). Dobell found spirochaetes in Indian grass snakes and described them as *Spirochaeta tropidonoti*. Scharrer (1935) found similar types in specimens of *Natrix natrix* L.

REFERENCES

Aronson, J. D. (1929). Spontaneous tuberculosis in snakes. *Arch. Path.* **8**, 159.

Boycott, R. S., Taylor, J. and Douglas, S. H. (1953). *Salmonella* in tortoises. *J. Path. Bact.* **65**, 401–411.

Breed, R. S., Murray, E. G. D. and Hitchens, A. F. (1927). *In* Bergey's "Manual of Determinative Bacteriology", 7th edn. Baltimore.

Brison, I., Tysset, C. and Vacher, F. B. (1959). Recherches sur les Pseudomonaceae. *Ann. Inst. Pasteur* **96**, 633.

Burtscher, J. (1931). Ueber die Mundfäule des Schlangen. *Zool. Garten* **4**, 235–244.

Buxton, A. (1957). "Salmonellosis in Animals." Farnham Royal, Bucks.

Caldwell, N. E. and Ryerson, D. L. (1940). A new species of the genus *Pseudomonas* pathogenic for certain reptiles. *J. Bact.* **39**, 323–336.

Camin, J. (1948). Mite transmission of a haemorrhagic septicaemia in snakes. *J. Parasit.* **34**, 345–354.

Clausen, H. J. and Durand-Reynals, F. (1937). Studies on the experimental infection of some reptiles, amphibia and fish with *Serratia anolium*. *Amer. J. Path.* **13**, 441–451.

Conti, L. F. and Crowley, J. H. (1939). A new bacterial species, isolated from the Chuckawalla (*Sauromalus varius*). *J. Bact.* **33**, 647–653.

Dobell, C. (1910). On some parasitic protozoa from Ceylon. *Spolia zeylanica* **3**, 78.

Graham-Jones, O. (1961). Notes on the common tortoise. *Vet. Rec.* **73**, 313–321.

Griffith, A. S. (1930). Tuberculosis in cold-blooded animals. *In* "A System of Bacteriology in relation to Medicine." Vol. *v*, 326–332.

Hunt, T. J. (1957). Notes on diseases and mortality in Testudines. *Herpetologica* **13**, 19–23.

Jaksztien, K. P. and Petzold, H. G. (1959). Durch *Salmonella* Infektion bedingte Schwierigkeiten bei der Aufzucht von Schlangen und ihre Behandlung. *Bl. Aqu. Terrk.* **6**, 79–80.

Kiesewetter, J., Rudat, K. D. and Seidel, G. (1960). Salmonellen und Reptilien. *Zbl. Bak.* I. Orig. **180**, 503–509.

Patrick, R. and Werkman, C. H. (1930). Notes on the bacterial flora of the snake. *Proc. Iowa Acad. Sci.* **37**, 330.

Rautlin de la Roy, Y. (1960). Révision taxonomique et intérêt en pathologie des bactéries gram-négatifs à pigments jaunes. Thesis for the degree of M.D. Univ. Toulouse, France, p. 89.

Reinhard, W. (1927). Ueber die Mundfäule der Schlangen. *Bl. Aqu. Terrk.* 318–321.

Scharrer, B. (1935). Ueber *Spirochaeta* (*Treponema*) *minutum* Dobell bei Amphibien. *Zool. Anz.* **111**, 1–7.

Willis, R. A. (1932). A bacillary disease of the blue-tongued lizard (*Tiliqua scincoides*). *Med. J. Austr.* **19**, 144–157.

B.   PROTOZOAL DISEASES

Flagellata

Flagellates (unicellular organisms, equipped with a whip or flagellum) may be found in the blood or in the fluid contents of the gut of reptiles. Among the blood parasites trypanosomes are most frequently encountered. They are comparatively large and similar to those seen in birds.

In terrestrial reptiles the trypanosomes are commonly transmitted by insects (Diptera), probably also by mites (Acarina). In aquatic forms the transmission takes place through the sucking activities of leeches (Hirudinea). The degree to which trypanosomiasis damages the health of an infected reptile depends probably on the severity of the infection.

Trypanosoma grayi Novy, which occurs in the blood of African crocodiles, has been extensively studied (Fig. 292 g–n). The developmental cycle of this parasite is well known because it relies, as intermittent host on the tsetse fly (*Glossina palpalis*) which transmits sleeping sickness in man. The length of *T. gràyi*—including flagella— may reach 91 μ. The body shows longitudinal stripes. Reproduction has so far only been observed to take place in the transmitting flies. According to Hoare (1931) it takes place in the mid-gut of the insect. In the end-gut young trypanosoma of 12–20 μ can be found. These are excreted with the faeces of the fly. It is assumed that flies are either accidentally squashed in the mouth of the crocodile or that they defaecate there.

Trypanosoma varani Wenyon has been found in various species of *Varanus*. It is transmitted by the fly *Glossina tachinoides* Westwood. The Indian gecko *Hemidactylus frenatus* Schlegel suffers from *Trypanosoma phlebotomi* Mackie transmitted by *Phlebotomus babu* var. *shorti* Adler and Theodor (Short and Swaminath, 1931). The authors, studying the reproductive phase of this parasite in the gut of the *Phlebotomus* fly reported the appearance of spherical cysts containing trypanosomes without flagella similar to *Leishmania* types. These divide and change into the "crithidial" form.

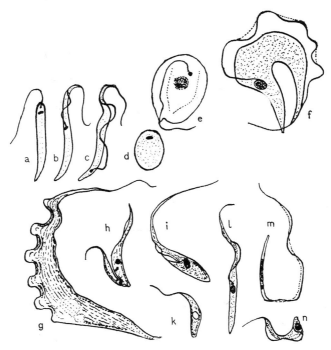

Fig. 292. Trypanosomes from reptiles. a, *Leptomonas*; b, *Crithidia*; c, *Trypanosoma*; d, Leishmania type. (From Reichenow, 1953.) e, *Trypanosoma platydactyli* Carr. × 1 600; f, *Trypanosoma martini* Bouet. × 1 000. (From Hoare.) g–n, *Trypanosoma grayi* Novy; g, From the blood of a crocodile; h–n, from the intestine of *Glossina palpalis* Rob.-Desv.; l–n, *Crithidia*. (After Hoare from Doflein-Reichenow, 1953.)

Further species of *Trypanosoma* have been described from the African gecko *Tarentola mauretanica* L., from *Chamaeleo vulgaris* L. from the Sudan, and from the Central African skink *Mabuya raddoni* Gray. The skinks *Mabuya maculilabris* Gray and *Mabuya striata* Peters harbour *Trypanosoma martini* Bouet; other types are *T. platydactyli* Catouillard, *T. chamaeleonis* Wenyon and *T. boueti* Martin.

Trypanosomes have also been found in the blood of various snakes. Reichenow (1953) mentions:

> *Trypanosoma erythrolampri* Wenyon from *Erythrolamprus aesculapii* L. one of the South American "false coral snakes";
>
> *Trypanosoma najae* Wenyon from *Naja nigricollis* Reinh., the black-necked cobra from the Sudan;
>
> *Trypanosoma clozeli* Bouet from *Tropidonotus ferox*, a grass snake;
>
> *Trypanosoma primeti* Mathis and Léger from *Natrix piscator* Schn., a S.E. Asian adder;
>
> *Trypanosoma brazili* Brumpt from *Helicops modestus* Gthr., a Brazilian aquatic snake. (Intermediate hosts: the leeches *Placobdella brasiliensis* and *Placobdella catenigera*.)

The same author lists the following species of *Trypanosoma* as occurring in tortoises:

> *Trypanosoma vittatus* Robertson from *Lissemys punctata granosa* (Schoepff) from Ceylon. The parasite is up to 70 μ long and is transmitted by a species of *Glossiphonia;*
>
> *Trypanosoma damoniae* Laveran and Mesnil from *Chinemys reevesii* Gray;
>
> *Trypanosoma pontyi* Bouet from *Pelusios subniger* Lac;
>
> *Trypanosoma chelodina* Johnson from *Chelodinia longicollis* Shaw.

The more primitive types of the trypanosomids are also commonly seen in reptiles, particularly the genus *Leptomonas* which lacks the undulating membrane typical of the higher forms. Quoting from the literature, particularly from Reichenow (1953) we find:

> *Leptomonas chamaeleonis* Wenyon in the gut of Chamaeleontidae;
>
> *Leptomonas* sp. in the gut and the blood of *Anolis* and *Chalcides ocellatus* Forsk.;
>
> *Leptomonas* sp. in *Agama stellio* L. (in the blood only) (Hindle, 1930);
>
> *Leptomonas* sp. in the gut of *Cnemidophorus lemniscatus*.

The type *Leishmania* which is spherical and lacks a flagella has been found in the blood of several lizards. Reichenow (1953) lists:

> *Leishmania tarentolae* Wenyon from *Tarentola mauretanica* L.;
>
> *Leishmania hemidactyli* Mackie *et al.* from the Indian *Hemidactylus gleadovii* Murray;
>
> *Leishmania ceramodactyli* Adler and Theodor from the oriental *Ceramodactylus doriae*;
>
> *Leishmania agamae*;

Leishmania adleri Heisch from *Latastia longicauda revoili* Vaillant (Heisch, 1958).

Heisch gave a detailed description of this species. Apart from typical *Leishmania* types he found many of the more primitive *Leptomonas* stages. The *Leishmania* parasites are transmitted by *Phlebotomus* flies.

The Bodonidae occur in their majority free-living in slightly saprobic waters. Some species appear occasionally or permanently as parasitic

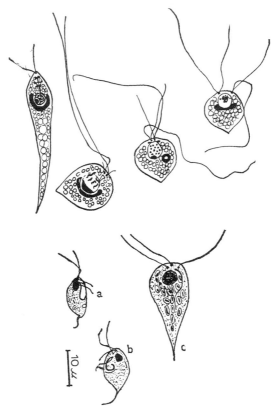

Fig. 293. *Bodonidae* from reptiles. Above: *Proteromonas lacertae-viridis* Grassi. (After Belar from Reichenow, 1953.) Left, resting form, right, reproductive stages. × 1 600. Below: a and b, *Chilomastix wenyoni* Janakidevi. c, *Chilomastix caulleryi* Alexeieff. × 1 000.

forms, both in the blood and in the intestine. *Proteromonas lacertae viridis* Grassi, which belongs to this group, is frequently found in the gut of lizards. It is a slender, pear-shaped protozoon with two flagella of 10–30 μ length (Fig. 293). It reproduces by longitudinal or multiple division within so-called pseudocysts. Chatton described a similar type from *Tarentola mauretanica* as var. *tarentolae*.

Proteromonas uromastixi from *Uromastix hardwicki* Gray was described by Janakidevi (1961).

The genus *Chilomastix* is distinguished by having three anterior and one posterior flagella. Reichenow (1953) saw a small type, not described in detail, in lizards and Janakidevi described a closely allied type *Retortomonas cheloni* in tortoises (1962) (Fig. 293).

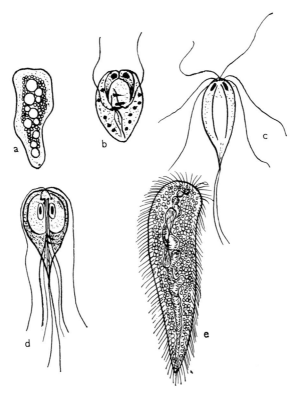

FIG. 294. a, *Vahlkampfia ranarum* Epstein and Ilowaisky. × 666. (From Reichenow.) b, *Trepomonas agilis* Duj. × 1 333. (After Bishop from Reichenow, 1953.) c, *Hexamita intestinalis* Duj. × 2 000. (From Reichenow, 1953.) d, *Lamblia microti* Kofoid and Christiansen. (From Reichenow, 1953.) e, *Protoopalina intestinalis* Stein. (After Metcalf from Reichenow, 1953.) (Note the long, excretory organelle.)

The genus *Vahlkampfia*, which has no flagella and has the shape of an oblong amoeba, is very occasionally seen in the reptilian intestine. Reichenow mentions *Vahlkampfia dobelli* Hartmann from *Lacerta muralis* L. and *Vahlkampfia reynoldsi* McFall from *Sceloporus undulatus* Latr. (see Wood, 1953).

Hexamita, a flagellate with eight flagella, usually found in fish and amphibians, can occasionally invade the intestine of chelonians. Alexeieff assigned these forms to a new species *Octomastix parvus*, which is not generally accepted as valid. Among other authors Lavier (1942) described *Hexamita* from chelonians (Fig. 294). Occasionally the parasite invades the circulatory system. Possibly identical with the free-living form is the related *Trepomonas agilis* Duj., equally equipped with eight flagella (Das Gupta, 1935) (Fig. 294).

Lamblia varani Lavier is a rare intestinal parasite from *Varanus niloticus* L. It is distinguished by a well-defined dorsal and ventral side, equipped with four pairs of flagella, and forms spherical cysts.

The genus *Trichomonas* too occurs parasitic in reptiles. *Monocercomonas colubrorum* Hammerschmidt is a commonly seen protozoon inhabiting the gut of lizards and snakes (Fig. 296a). Grassé (1926) considers this parasite, which has three posterior flagella, as identical with several other flagellates, described as *Trichomastix lacertae* Blochmann; *T. viperae* Léger; *T. serpentis* Dobell; *T. mabuiae* Dobell; and *T. saurii* Da Fonseca. The genus has, on occasion, been found to invade the blood stream of reptilians.

Das Gupta (1930) described a similar type of *Trichomonas*, found in the intestine of a chameleon, as *"Eutrichomastix"*. The exact species was not determined (Fig. 296c).

Monocercomonoides varies from *Monocercomonas* by the fact that the flagella issue in pairs from two basal bodies. The axillary rod is slender. *M. lacertae* Tanabe occurs in the rectum of the lizard *Eremias arguta* Pallas (Reichenow, 1953). *M. filamentum* Janakidevi (1961) was found in chelonians. Honigberg (1935) reported an investigation of the related genus *Hexamastix* and found the species *H. kirby* and *H. crassus* in *Sauromalus obesus* Baird and *Eumeces gilberti* van Denburgh (Fig. 295c, d).

In 1961 Janakidevi found two further species, *Hexamastix lacertae*, an intestinal parasite of *Uromastix hardwicki* Gray, and *Hexamastix dobelli* which occurs in *Testudo elegans* Schoepff (Fig. 295e). Both authors demonstrate in their illustrations the great variability of these species.

Occasionally the related genus *Tritrichomonas* may be met with. *T. lacertae* Prowazek inhabits the cloaca of several lizards (Fig. 296d), *T. boae* Reichenow was found in *Constrictor constrictor* L. The latter species has three anterior and one posterior flagella; the posterior one forms the edge of an undulating membrane which connects it with the body of the flagellate. In *Tritrichomonas lacertae* we find three anterior

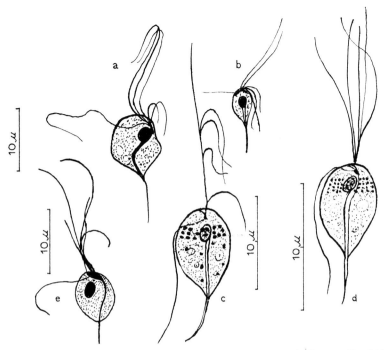

FIG. 295. Trichomonadina from reptiles. a and b, *Hexamastix lacertae* Janakidevi; c, *Hexamastix kirby* Honigberg; d, *Hexamastix crassus* Honigberg; e, *Hexamastix dobelli* Janakidevi. (a, b, and c, after Janakidevi; c and d, after Honigberg.)

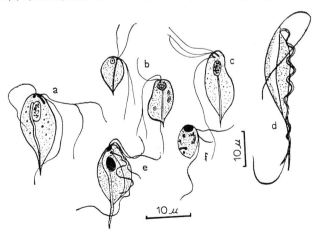

FIG. 296. a, *Monocercomonas colubrorum* Hammerschmidt. × 1 000. (After v. Prowazek from Reichenow, 1953.) b, *Tritrichomonas alexeieffi* Grassé. c, "*Eutrichomastix*" (= *Monocercomonas*) sp. from a chameleon. (From Das Gupta.) d, *Tritrichomonas lacertae* Prowazek. (After Grassé.) e, *Tritrichomonas lissemyi* Janakidevi. f, *Alexeiefella cheloni* Janakidevi.

flagella of equal length, whereas those of *T. boae* are of unequal length. Some similar types found in *Natrix natrix* L. and in *Python molurus* have not been described in detail. Grassé (1926) described *Tritrichomonas alexeieffi* from the rectum of the slow-worm (*Anguis fragilis* L.) and Janakidevi (1961) from that of *T. lissemyi* (Fig. 295e).

One group of trichomonads is described as *Trichocercomitus* (formerly *"Trimitus"*). Saxe and Schmidt found *T. parvus* in snakes and *T. trionyci* Knowles and Gupta in chelonians. Janakidevi determined a similar parasite, found in the Indian *Lissemys punctata granosa* Schoepff, as *Alexeiefella cheloni* (Fig. 296f).

Some Reptilia harbour representatives of the genus *Trichomonas* which is equipped with four anterior flagella. Alexeieff (1911) found *Trichomonas brumpti* in the chelonians *Nicoria* and *Testudo*, Parasi (quoted after Reichenow, 1953) discovered a trichomonad in *Crocodilus palustris* Lesson which he took to be *T. provazeki* A., an intestinal parasite of amphibians. Das Gupta (1936) found unknown species of *Trichomonas* in the Indian snake *Liopeltis calamaria* Gthr. and in the N. American snake *Natrix erythrogaster*.

The flagellate genus *Opalina*, so commonly seen in frogs, may occasionally also be encountered in saurians. Lavier (1927) reports on finding *Protoopalina nyanzae* Lavier in *Varanus niloticus* from Lake Victoria. Carini (1943) found *Zelleriella* spp. in Brazilian snakes but considered them as derived from frogs eaten by the snakes.

Rhizopoda

Amoebae seem to be more common parasites in reptiles than in amphibians. *Entamoeba invadens* Rodhain is known to cause losses among lizards and snakes (Geiman and Ratcliffe, 1936). The species proved harmless to mammals. Morphologically it closely resembles *Entamoeba histolytica* Schaudinn, which plays such an important part in human pathology. Like the latter species *E. invadens* produced the clinical picture of membranous enteritis. There are recent reports (Hill, 1953) from the London Zoo about the ravages caused by this rhizopod in lizards and snakes. The affected gut becomes inflamed and oedematous. The inflammation gives cause to peritoneal adhesions. The intestinal mucosa becomes ulcerated, the parasite invades the submucosa and reaches the liver by way of the portal vein. Massive infarction occurs in the liver and the affected animal dies. Figure 297 shows various stages in the development of the parasite in a case of ulcerative colitis.

Steck (1962), investigating the amoebic dysentery of snakes, found them suffering from haemorrhagic colitis with much cellular damage and subsequent necrosis caused, perhaps, by the effects of a toxic colonic flora. Amoebic invasion of the liver produced foci of thrombosis and necrobiosis.

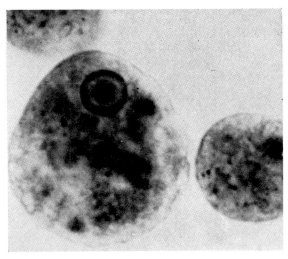

Fig. 297. *Entamoeba invadens* Rodhain from ulcerations in the colon of an aquatic snake *Natrix rhombifera* Hallowell. × 1 600. (After Ratcliffe from Schlumberger in Cohrs, Jaffé and Meesen, 1958.)

Reichenow (1953) mentions the following types of *Entamoeba* as occurring in reptilians:

Entamoeba varani Lavier from *Varanus niloticus* L. (perhaps identical with *E. invadens*?);

E. lacerticola Wood from various lizards (Wood, 1933);

E. terrapenae Sanders and Cleveland from *Pseudemys scripta elegans* Wieg.;

E. insolita Geiman and Wichterman from *Testudo elephantina* Harlan;

E. barreti Taliaferro and Holmes (cysts with eight nuclei as against four in *terrapenae* and *insolita*) from *Chelydra serpentina* L.;

E. flaviviridis Knowles and Das Gupta (similar to the last mentioned) from *Hemidactylus flaviviridis* Rüpp.;

E. spec. in *Lacerta* spp. and in *Agama stellio* L.;

E. testudinis Hartmann (size up to 70 μ; no cysts seen) from *Testudo graeca* L. and from other terrestrial tortoises;

E. serpentis Cunha and Fonseca (no cysts seen) from the snake *Drimobius bifossatus* Radday.

Sporozoa

Sporozoal infections are comparatively common in reptilians and are mostly due either to intestinal infection of the gut with *Eimeria* or to *Plasmodia* invading the blood.

Sub-class Telosporidia

In spite of assertions to the contrary the Order Gregarinida have not definitely been proved to be pathogenic for Reptilia. Schöppler (1917) who found Gregarinida in *Lacerta agilis* L. thought that they had gained access through mealworms used for feeding the lizards.

Order Coccidia
Sub-order Adeleidea

Karyolysus lacertae Danilewsky is a haemoparasite of lizards which requires an intermediate host. It is found in the endothelial lining of blood vessels of *Lacerta muralis* L. where it reproduces asexually. Sexual reproduction takes place in the mite *Neoliponyssus saurarum* Oudemans. The merozoite, having gained access to the blood of the lizard, surrounds itself with a membrane and divides into 8–30 macromerozoites. They immigrate into new endothelial cells where, in turn, they again grow to schizonts. Eventually two types of schizonts of different sizes appear: macro- and micromerozoites (Fig. 298a). They invade the erythrocytes of the lizard and form a capsule. Further development can only take place in the next host, the mite. If *Neoliponyssus* sucks up infected blood the encapsulated sexual forms are freed and are now easily distinguished as broad macro- and slender microgametes. A pair of these adhere closely to one another, penetrate an intestinal mucosal cell, and surround themselves with a membrane. The macrogamete grows; the microgamete divides. One of the microgametes fertilizes the macrogamete which now grows into a large oocyst. The oocyst disintegrates into filariform sporokinetes which in their turn invade the eggs of the acarid. Here they change into spores which eventually divide into 20–30 sporozoites. If the lizard feeds on infected acarid nymphs the sporozoites or merozoites gain access to the intestinal canal and the circle is repeated. These merozoites are very motile and move across the intestinal epithelium until they gain access to a capillary vessel.

The deleterious effect of this infection rests mainly on the deformation or fragmentation, rarely in the complete destruction of the erythrocyte nucleus.

The number of *Karyolysus* species pathogenic for reptiles is probably large. Few, however, have been as thoroughly studied as *K. lacertae*.

Mixed infections are also likely to occur. Among other species of *Karyolysus* which develop in acarids we may mention *K. bicapsulatus*

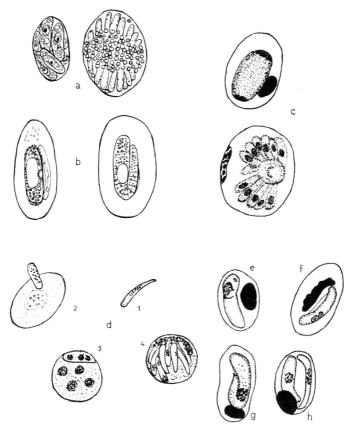

FIG. 298. Adeleidea from reptiles. a, *Karyolysus lacertae* Danilewsky. × 666. (From Reichenow, 1953.) b, *Karyolysus bicapsulatus* Franca. × 1 200. (From Reichenow, 1953.) c, *Hepatozoon pettiti* Thiroux. (From Hoare.) d, *Haemogregarina stepanovi* Danilewsky. 1, Infectious sporozoite; 2, schizont, penetrating the erythrocyte of a tortoise; 3, syncarion in the process of dividing, with three remaining microgametes; 4, eight sporozoites. (From Reichenow, 1953.) e, *Haemogregarina musotae* Hoare. f, *Haemogregarina enswerae* Hoare. g, *Haemogregarina sternothaeri* Hoare. h, *Haemogregarina crotaphopeltis* Hoare. (e–h, After Hoare.)

Franca (Fig. 298b) from *Lacerta muralis* L. and *K. zuluetai* Reichenow from the same host. The species *K. lacazei* Labbé from *Lacerta viridis* Laur., *Lacerta ocellata* Daud. and *Psammodromus algirus* L. develop not in the ovary but in the peritoneal cavity of the mite.

It is difficult to distinguish the various species of *Karyolysus* from one another. The capsules containing the gametocytes of *K. bicapsulatus* and *K. zuluetai* for example are recognized by a polar reinforcement which has been likened to a skull-cap. *K. lacazei* is distinguished as having large gametocytes which assume a curved shape in the erythrocytes (Fig. 298b).

The genus *Hepatozoon* is closely related to *Karyolysus*. It differs in the fact that the oocyst does not produce sporokinetes but numerous spores containing sporozoites (Fig. 298c). Like *Karyolysus, Hepatozoon* invades the erythrocytes and a change of host takes place between reptile and arthropod. Hoare (1933) found various stages of schizogony and sexual types in erythrocytes of *Crocodilus niloticus* Laur. the parasite being *Hepatozoon pettiti* Thiroux. Sporogony stages were also found in the peritoneal cavity of the tsetse fly *Glossina palpalis* Rob.-Desv. Actual stages of copulation could not be observed but the author succeeded in transmitting the disease experimentally from the fly to the crocodile.

The intestinal submucosa, the lung and the liver of *Gecko verticillatus* has been found infected with *Hepatozoon mesnili*. Oocysts and sporozoites were found in *Culex fatigans* Wied. Another invader of erythrocytes, *Hepatozoon mauretanicum*, was found in chelonians (*Testudo graeca* L.). *Hepatozoon mauretanicum* Sergent is thought to be transmitted by the acarid *Hyalomma aegyptium* (*syriacum*), a mite which is frequently found attached to tortoises imported as pets (Arthur, 1963). In the case of *Hepatozoon triatomae* Osimani which parasitizes the lizard *Tupinambis teguixin* L. infectious spores have been found in the peritoneal cavity of the bug *Triatoma rubrovaria* Pinto.

The genus *Haemogregarina*, the oocyst of which produces 8 sporozoites without producing spores first, has been found in snakes and tortoises. Leeches function as intermediate hosts. While they are sucking blood from the reptiles young sporozoites gain access to the circulatory system and invade erythrocytes (Fig. 298e). Gametes may be found in the red blood corpuscles of the leech (Fig. 298e–g). Conjugation of the macrogamete with one of the four available microgametes takes place in the intestinal epithelium; finally eight sporozoites develop from a synkarion and these gain access to the proboscis of the leech. *Haemogregarina stepanovi* Danilewsky from *Emys orbicularis* L. is transmitted by *Haementeria costata* (Müller). The lungs of the Indian tortoise *Geomyda trijuga* (Schweigg) are occasionally invaded by *Haemogregarina castellani* Wiley, the leech *Ozobranchus shipleyi* serving as intermediate host.

Hoare (1932) made extensive investigations of haemogregarines in snakes and tortoises of East Africa and established the following species:

Haemogregarina rubirizi Hoare, from *Mehelya capensis savergnani*;

H. musotae Hoare, from *Boaedon lineatus* Dum. and Bib. (Fig. 298e);

H. crotaphopeltis Hoare, from *Crotaphopeltis hotamboeia* Laur. (Fig. 298h);

H. enswerae Hoare, from *Naja melanoleuca* Schl. (Fig. 298f);

H. sternothaeri Hoare, from the tortoise *Pelusios sinuatus* Smith (Fig. 298g).

Figs. 298e–h, which are taken from C. A. Hoare's papers, reproduce some of the developmental stages of this parasite.

Sub-order Eimeriidea

Many members of this group are reptilian parasites. They are commonly found in the gut or the gall bladder, more rarely in the liver or the blood. There are usually no intermediate hosts, only *Schellackia* passes a part of its development in acarids. Systematically the group is distinguished by the fact that macro- and microgametes develop separately. Genera are distinguished by the number of the final sporozoites into *Eimeria, Globidium, Isospora, Cyclospora, Caryospora, Tyzzeria, Wenyonella* and *Schellackia*. While *Eimeria* develops four spores, each with two sporozoites, *Isospora* develops two spores with four sporozoites each; *Cyclospora* two spores, each with two sporozoites; *Caryospora* one spore containing eight sporozoites; and *Wenyonella* four spores with four sporozoites each. *Globidium* differs from *Eimeria* by causing the host cell to hypertrophy and by producing double-walled oocysts. *Tyzzeria* and *Caryospora* are similar in their morphology. For details the special literature, particularly Reichenow (1953), should be consulted.

Eimeriidea commonly found in reptiles are:

Eimeria railleti Léger in the intestine of the slow-worm (Lavier, 1938);

Eimeria geckonis Tanabe in the intestine of *Emys orbicularis* L.;

Eimeria mitraria Laveran and Mesnil in the intestine of the Asiatic turtle *Chinemys reevesii* Gray;

Eimeria tropidonoti Guyénot, Naville and Ponse from the intestine of *Natrix natrix* L. (Fig. 299a);

Eimeria legeri Simond from the gall bladder of the Indian *Lissemys punctata granosa* Schoepff.;

Eimeria agamae Laveran and Pettit in the bile of *Agama agama* L.;

Eimeria scinci Phisalix in the bile of *Scincus officinalis* L.;

Eimeria flaviviridis Setna and Bana in the bile of *Hemidactylus flaviviridis* Rüpp. (Fig. 299b);

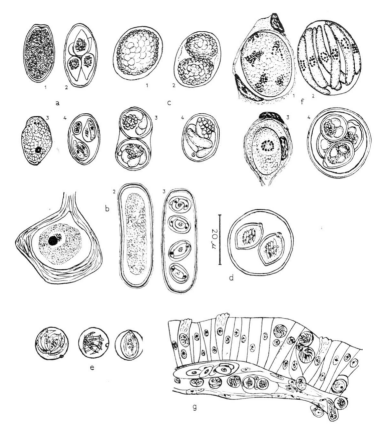

Fig. 299. Eimeriidea from reptiles. a, *Eimeria tropidonoti* Guyénot, Naville and Ponse. × 725. 1, oocyst; 2, sporoblasts; 3, macrogamete; 4, oocyst with spores. (After Guy. Nav. and Ponse.) b, *Eimeria flaviviridis* Setna and Bana. c, *Isospora dirumpens* Hoare. 1, oocyst; 2, oocyst with sporoblasts; 3, sporocysts; 4, mature sporocyst. (From Hoare.) d, *Isospora xantusiae* Amrein; e, *Caryospora simplex* Léger. × 600. (From Reichenow, 1953.) f, *Wenyonella africana* Hoare. 1, Schizone; 2, merozoites; 3, macrogametocyst; 4, oocyst with spores. × 1 200. (After Hoare.) g, *Schellackia bolivari* Reichenow. (From Reichenow, 1953.)

Eimeria cystis-felleae Debaisieux in the bile of *Natrix natrix* L.;
Eimeria zaenuis Phisalix in *Coluber constrictor* L. (Roudabush);
Eimeria amydae Roudabush in *Amyda spinifer* Le Sueur;
Eimeria clericksoni Roudabush in *Amyda spinifer* Le Sueur;
Eimeria hermoganti Simond in the spleen of *Gavialis gangeticus* Gmel.;

Globidium navillei Harant and Cazal. Subepithelial in the gut of *Natrix natrix* L. and in *Natrix maura* L. (Harant and Cazal, 1954); *Isospora dirumpens* Hoare in *Bitis arietans* (Fig. 299c);

Isospora fragilis Léger in the intestine of *Vipera aspis* L.;

Isospora knowlesi Ray and Das Gupta in *Hemidactylus flaviviridis* Rüpp.;

Isospora mesnili Sergent in the gut of *Chamaeleo vulgaris* L.;

Isospora natricis Yakimoff and Gousseff in the gut of *Natrix natrix* L.;

Isospora phisalix Yakimoff and Gouseff in the gut of *Elaphe quatuor-lineata* Lac.;

Isospora xantusiae Amrein in the intestinal epithelium of *Xantusia vigilis* Baird and *Xantusia henshawi* Stejneger (Fig. 299d);

Cyclospora viperae Phisalix intestinal in French vipers and adders;

Cyclospora sp. in *Hemidactylus frenatus* Dum. and Bibr.;

Caryospora brasiliensis Carini in *Cobra* species;

Caryospora jararacae in *Bothrops jararaca* Wied.;

Caryospora legeri Hoare in *Psammophis sibilans* L.;

Caryospora simplex Léger intestinal in *Vipera aspis* L. (Fig. 299e);

Tyzzeria natrix Matubayasi in the Japanese *Natrix tigrina*;

Wenyonella africana Hoare, intestinal in the African snake *Boaedon lineatus* Dum. and Bibr. (Hoare, 1933) (Fig. 299f).

The genus *Dorisiella* resembles *Isospora* in producing two sporocysts, but while those of *Isospora* contain four sporozoites, those of *Dorisiella* contain eight. Yakimoff and Gouseff (1953) found, however, a type of *Dorisiella hoari* in an Italian species of *Elaps*, with four or six sporozoites. The systematic position of the genus therefore remains doubtful.

Fig. 299g shows the invasion of the intestinal mucosa of *Psammodromus hispanicus* Fitzinger and the presence of several stages of the eimerid *Schellackia bolivari* Reichenow. The parasite develops in the mid-gut of lizards. The sporozoites invade lymphocytes or erythrocytes and are eventually sucked up by the acarid *Neoliponyssus saurarum* Oudemans, which merely acts as a transmitting vehicle for the parasite. Lizards may also harbour a closely related eimerid, *Wenyonella minuta* Franca.

Sub-order Haemosporidia

Analogous to the well-known malaria parasite of man there are blood parasites in other mammalians, birds and reptiles. Most of the intermediate transmitting hosts are arthropods.

Haemoproteus tarentolae Riding occurs in the erythrocytes of geckos; *H. metchnikovi* Simond in the tortoise *Chitra indica* Gray. Similar types are listed by Reichenow (1953):

Haemoproteus simondi (Castellani and Viley from *Hemidactylus* spp.)
(Fig. 300);

H. grahami Shortt from *Agama nupta* de Filippi;

H. gonzalesi Iturbe from *Anolis biporcatus* Gray;

H. mesnili Bouet from African snakes (Fig. 300).

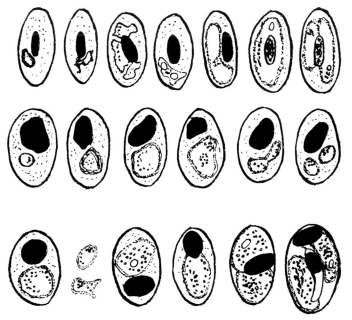

FIG. 300. Above: *Haemoproteus mesnili* Bouet. Approx. × 1 000. (After Macfie from Reichenow, 1953.) Middle and below: *Haemoproteus simondi* Castellani and Wiley. Approx. × 1 000. (From Dobell and Mühlens in Reichenow, 1953.)

Plasmodium (Family Plasmodiidae *Mesnil*) has so far only been seen in lizards. *Plasmodium minasense* Carini and Rudolph (Fig. 301, 1–6) from *Mabuia agilis* Radday, and *Goniocephalus borneensis* Schlegel (Laird, 1960) may serve as examples. *Plasmodium vastator* Laird has been seen in the flying lizard *Draco volans* Gray. The intermediate hosts of these parasites are as yet unknown.

Reichenow (1953) and Laird (1960) mention the further species of *Plasmodium* as occurring in reptilians:

Plasmodium agamae Wenyon in *Agama agama* L.;

P. diploglossi Arago and Neiva in *Diploglossus fasciatus* (Gray);

P. cnemidophori Carini in *Cnemidophorus lemniscatus* D.;

P. mabuiae Wenyon in *Mabuia quinquetaeniata* Sternfield;

P. maculilabre Schwetz in *Mabuia maculilabris* Gray;

P. pitmani Hoare in the same host and in *Mabuia striata* Peters;

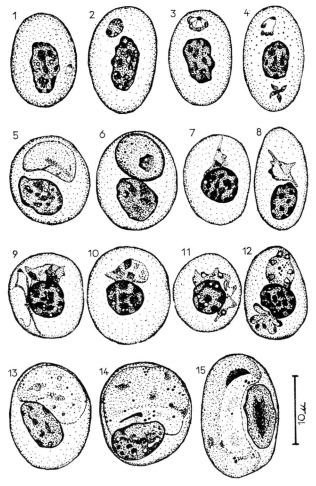

FIG. 301. 1–6. *Plasmodium minasense* Carini and Rudolph. × 1 900. (From Laird, 1960.) 7–15. *Plasmodium vastator* Laird. × 1 900. (From Laird, 1960.)

P. lacertiliae Thompson and Hart in *Leiolepisma fuscum* (D. & B.);

P. terrealbae Scorze and Dagert Boyer in *Anolis*;

P. pifanoi Scorze and Dagert Boyer in *Ameiva ameiva ameiva* L.;

P. lygosomae Laird in *Lygosoma moco* Gray;

P. tropiduri Aragao and Neiva in the Brazilian *Tropidurus torquatus*;

P. mexicanum Thompson and Huff in *Sceloporus ferrariperezi*;
P. rhadimurum Thompson and Huff, in *Iguana iguana* L. (Mexico);
P. floridense Thompson and Huff in *Sceloporus undulatus* Latr. (Florida).

Piroplasmida *Patton*

A brief mention should here be made of the *Piroplasmida*. The

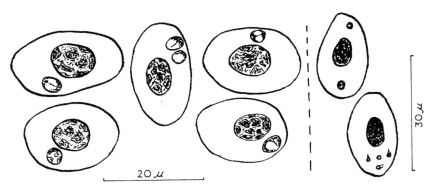

Fig. 302. Left: *Aegyptianella emydis*, a parasite of erythrocytes. (From Brumpt and Lavier.) Right: Another parasite of erythrocytes, *Nuttalia guglielmi* Carpano.

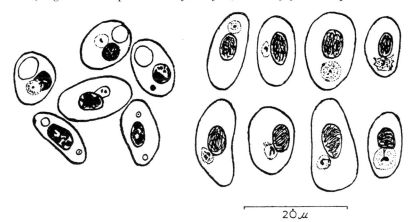

Fig. 303. Left: *Pirhemocyton tarentolae* Chatton and Blanc from *Tarentola mauretanica* L. (From Chatton and Blanc.) Right: *Pirhemocyton lacertae* Chatton and Blanc from *Lacerta viridis* L. (After Brumpt and Lavier.)

systematic position of the whole order or group is as yet uncertain. Carpano (1939) described *Nuttalia guglielmi*, a blood parasite of this group from the tortoise *Testudo marginata* (Fig. 302, right). *Sauroplasma thomasi* du Toit is reported as producing similar annular inclusions in the erythrocytes of the S. African *Cordylus giganteus* Smith. Brumpt and Lavier (1935) succeeded in experimental infections of *Lacerta viridis* L. with *Babesia pirhemocyton* Chatton and Blanc. They established *Pirhemocyton tarentolae* Chatton and Blanc from the gecko *Tarentola mauretanica* L. and the allied species *P. lacertae* Brumpt and Lavier (Fig. 303, right).

The same authors found piroplasmids in erythrocytes of *Clemmys caspica leprosa* Lov. and Williams. They called the parasite *Tunetella emydis* (Fig. 302, left). Carpano (1939) suggests the name of *Aegyptianella* for this genus, in which case the specific name should be changed to *Aegyptianella emydis*.

Sub-class Cnidosporidia

Few members of this sub-class, mostly Myxo- and Microsporidia, have been found in reptilians, among them the genera *Myxidium* and *Glugea*. Kudo (1919) found *Myxidium danilewskyi* Laveran in renal tubules of *Emys orbicularis* L., *Myxidium mackiei* Bosanquet in *Trionyx gangeticus* Cuv. and *Myxidium americanum* Kudo in *Trionyx spiniferus* Le Sueur.

The microsporidian *Glugea danilewskyi* Pfr. (Fig. 304) is described

  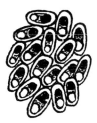

FIG. 304. *Glugea danilewskyi* Guyénot and Naville (probably a *Plistophora*). Left: Sporoblast with maturing spores. × 2 350. Right: Mature spores. × 4 700. (From Guyénot and Naville.)

from frogs, *Emys orbicularis* L. and from *Natrix natrix* (Danilewsky, 1891). Guyénot and Naville reported on the appearance of *Glugea ghigii* in snakes. *Glugea* has also occasionally been seen in trematodes infesting reptilians where they may serve as intermediate or transmitting hosts.

Sub-class Sarcosporidia

Sarcosporidia, well known from the muscle-fibres of mammals and birds, appear occasionally in reptiles in the form of small grey tubes containing spores. *Sarcocystis platydactyli* Bertram has been found in *Platydactylus mauretanicus*, *Sarcocystis gongyli* Trinci in *Chalcides ocellatus* Fors., *Sarcocystis lacertae* in *Lacerta muralis* L. and *Sarcocystis pythonis* Tiegs in *Python spilotes* (Tiegs, 1931).

Ciliata

The ciliates do not play a large part among the intestinal parasites of reptiles. Johnston and Amrein (1952) have drawn our attention to the genus *Nyctotherus*, a bean- or heart-shaped ciliate, uniformly covered with ciliary rows. It has a long, curved cytostom (Fig. 305). The species that may be encountered are in particular:

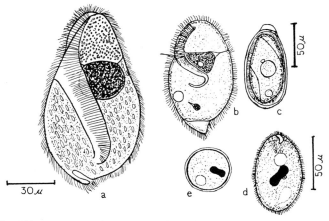

Fig. 305. Ciliates from reptiles. a, *Nyctotherus hardwickii* Ianakidevi; b, *Nyctotherus teleaceus* Geiman and Wichterman; c = b, encysted; d, *Balantidium testudinis* Chagas. e = d, encysted. (After Janakidevi. b–e, after Geiman and Wichterman.)

Nyctotherus haranti Grassé in *Tarentola mauretanica* L.;

N. *beltrani* Hegner in *Ctenosaurus acanthurus* Shaw;

N. *kyphodes* Geiman and Wichtermann from the tortoises *Testudo elephantopus hoodensis* van Denburgh and *Testudo vicina* Spix;

N. *teleacus* Geiman and Wichterman from the same host (Fig. 305b);

N. *woodi* Amrein from the Californian reptiles *Xanthusia vigilis* Baird, *Xanthusia henshawi* Stejneger, *Dipsosaurus dorsalis* B. and G. and *Sauromalus obesus*;

N. *sokoloffi* Schouten from *Amphisbaena albocingulata* Boettger;

N. *trachysauri* Johnston from *Trachysaurus rugosus* Gray;

N. *hardwickii* Janakidevi from *Uromastix hardwickii* Gray (Fig. 305c).

These ciliates usually populate the large intestine. They are not known to have any definite pathogenic effect and may be simple symbionts.

The same may be said of the closely related genus *Balantidium* which Geiman and Wichtermann (1937) found in the Galapagos tortoise *Testudo elephantopus hoodensis* van Denburgh (Fig. 305d). The authors described the species as *Balantidium testudinis* Chagas. Both this and the closely related species *Nyctotheruš teleaceus* as well as *N. kyphodes* and *N. woodi* Amrein have a tendency to form cysts (Fig. 305c and e).

REFERENCES

Alexeieff, A. (1911). Notes sur les Flagellées. *Arch. Zool. exp.* gen. ser. 5, **6**, 491–527.

Amrein, Y. U. (1952a). A new species of *Isopora*, *I. xantusiae* from S. Calif. lizards. *J. Parasit.* **38**, 147–150.

Amrein, Y. U. (1952b). A new species of *Nyctotherus*, *N. woodi* from S. Calif. lizards. *J. Parasit.* **38**, 266–270.

Arthur, D. R. (1963). "British Ticks." Butterworths, London.

Brumpt, E. and Lavier, G. (1935). Sur un Hématozoaire nouveau du. Lézard vert, *Pirhemocyton lacertae* n. sp. *Ann. Parasit. hum. comp.* **13**, 537–543.

Brumpt, E. and Lavier, G. (1935b). Sur un Piroplasmide nouveau, parasite de Tortue *Tunetella emydis* n. g. n. sp. *Ann. Paiasit. hum. comp.* **13**, 544–550.

Carini, A. (1943). Novas observacones en batraquios e ofidios, de zelleriellas hiperparasitadas por entamebas. *Arqu. Biol. S. Paulo* **27**, No. 255, 64–68.

Carpano, M. (1939). Sui piroplasmidi dei cheloni e sua una nuova specie rinvenuta nelle tartarhuge *Nuttallia guglielmi. Riv. parasit.* **3**, 267–276.

Danilewsky, B. (1891). Ueber die Myoparasiten der Amphibien und Reptilien. *Zbl. Bakt.* **9**, 9–10.

Das Gupta, B. M. (1935). The occurrence of a *Trepomcnas* sp. in the caecum of turtles. *J. Parasit.* **21**, 125–126.

Das Gupta, B. M. (1936). *Trichomonas* from the gut contents of a coral snake. *Parasitology* **28**, 202–205.

Das Gupta, B. M. (1936). Observations on the flagellates of the genera *Trichomonas* and *Eutrichomastix. Parasitology* **28**, 195–201.

Geiman, Q. M. and Ratcliffe, H. L. (1936). Morphology and life cycle of an amoeba producing amoebiasis in reptiles. *Parasitology* **28**, 208–228.

Geiman, Q. M. and Wichterman, R. (1937). Intestinal protozoa from Galapagos tortoises with description of three new species. *J. Parasit.* **23**, 331–347.

Grassé, P. (1926). Contribution à l'étude des flagellées parasites. *Arch. Zool. exp.* **65**, 345–602.

Guyénot, E. and Naville, A. (1922). Recherches sur le parasitisme et l'évolution d'une microsporidie, *Glugea danilewskyi* Pfr. (?) parasite de la couleuvre. *Rev. suisse Zool.* **30**, 1–62.

Guyénot, E. and Naville, A. (1924). *Glugea encyclometrae* n. sp. et *G. ghigii* n.sp. parasites de platodes et leur développement dans l'hôte vertébré *Tropidonotus natrix* L. *Rev. suisse Zool.* **31**, 75–115.

Harant, H. and Cazal, P. (1934). Remarques sur le genre *Globidium: Globidium navillei* n. sp. parasite de la couleuvre. *Ann. Parasit. hum. comp.* **12**, 162–169.

Hegner, R. (1940). *Nyctotherus beltrani* n. sp., a ciliate from an iguana. *J. Parasit.* **26**, 315–317.

Hegner, R. and Hewitt, R. (1940). A new genus and new species of amoeba from Mexican lizards. *J. Parasit.* **26**, 319–321.

Heisch, R. B. (1958). On *Leishmania adleri* sp. nov. from lacertid lizards (*Latastia* sp.) in Kenya. *Ann. trop. Med.* **52**, 68–72.

Hewitt, R. (1940). *Haemoproteus metchnikovi* Simond, 1901 from the yellow-bellied terrapin *Pseudemys elegans. Ann. trop. Med.* **52**, 273–278.

Hill, W. C. O. (1953). An epizootic due to *Entamoeba invadens* at the Garden of the Zoological Society. *Proc. zool. Soc. Lond.* **123**, 731–737.

Hindle, E. (1930). Attempts to infect hamsters with various flagellates. *Trans. roy. Soc. trop. Med.* **24**, 97–104.

Hoare, C. A. (1931). Studies on *Trypanosoma grayi*. III. Life cycle in the tsetse fly and in the crocodile. *Parasitology* **23**, 449–484.

Hoare, C. A. (1932). On protozoal blood parasites, collected in Uganda, with an account of the life cycle of the crocodile haemogregarine. *Parasitology* **24**, 210–224.

Hoare, C. A. (1933). Studies on some ophidian and avian coccidia from Uganda with a revision of the classification of the *Eimeridae. Parasitology* **25**, 359–388.

Honigberg, B. M. (1955). Structure and morphogenesis of two new species of *Hexamastix* from Liberia. *J. Parasit.* **41**, 1–17.

Ippen, R. (1959). Die Amoebendysenterie der Reptilien. *Kleintierpraxis* **4**, 131–137.

Janakidevi, K. (1961a). A new species of *Chilomastix* Alexeieff 1912. (Protozoa. Retortomonadines Grassé 1952) from the Indian lizard. *Z. Parasitenk.* **20**, 563–567.

Janakidevi, K. (1961b). A new species of *Hexamastix* (Protozoa) parasitic in the spiny-tailed lizard *Uromastix hardwicki. Z. Parasitenk.* **21**, 151–154.

Janakidevi, K. (1961c). A new ciliate from the spiny-tailed lizard. *Z. Parasitenk.* **21**, 155–158.

Janakidevi, K. (1961d). A new species of *Proteromonas* from the spiny-tailed lizard. *Arch. Protistenk.* **105**, 450–454.

Janakidevi, K. (1961e). *Hexamastix dobelli* n. sp. a new Trichomonad, parasitic in the starred tortoise. *J. Protozool.* **8**, 294–296.

Janakidevi, K. (1961f). Description of a new protozoon, *Alexieffella cheloni* n. gen. n. sp. *Ann. Mag. Nat. Hist.* Ser. 13. **IV**, 192–202.

Janakidevi, K. (1961g). The morphology of *Monocercomonoides filamentum* n. sp., parasite of the Indian starred tortoise. *Arch. Protistenk.* **106**, 37–40.

Janakidevi, K. (1961h). *Tritrichomonas lissemyi* n. sp., a parasite protozoon from the turtle. *Ann. Mag. Nat. Hist.* Ser. 13. **IV**, 411–414.

Janakidevi, K. (1961i). On *Retortomonas cheloni* n. sp., a parasitic protozoon from the starred tortoise. *Parasitology* **52**, 165–168.

Johnston, T. H. (1932). The parasites of the "stumpy tail" lizard *Trachysaurus rugosus. Trans. Roy. Soc. Austr.* **56**, 62–70.

Knowles, R. G. and Gupta, B. M. D. (1930). On two intestinal protozoa of an Indian turtle. *Indian J. med. Res.* **18**, 97–104.

Kudo, R. (1919). "Studies on Myxosporidia." Illinois Biol. Monographs, Vol. 5, 3 and 4.

Laird, M. (1951). *Plasmodium lygosomae* n. sp., a parasite of a New Zealand skink, *Lygosoma moco* Gray. *J. Parasit.* **37**, 183–189.

Laird, M. (1960). Malayan Protozoa. 3. Saurian malaria parasites. *J. Protozool.* **7**, 245–250.

Lavier, G. (1927). *Protoopalina nyanza* n. sp., opaline parasite d'un reptile. *C.R. Soc. Biol., Paris* **97**, 1709–1710.

Lavier, G. (1938). Sur *Eimeria raillieti* Léger 1899, coccidie intestinale d'*Anguis fragilis*. *Ann. Parasit. hum. comp.* **16**, 215–219.

Lavier, G. (1942). Sur une localisation atypique du parasitisme dans le genre *Hexamita*. *C.R. Soc. Biol., Paris* **136**, 20–22.

Reichenow, E. (1953). "Lehrbuch der Protozoenkunde." (Doflein-Reichenow), 6th edn., Fischer, Jena.

Rodhain, J. and van Hoof, M. Th. (1935). Sur le rôle pathogène d'*Entamoeba invadens*. *C. R. Soc. Biol., Paris* **118**, 1646–1650.

Roudabush, R. L. (1937). Some Coccidia of reptiles found in N. America. *J. Parasit.* **23**, 345–359.

Saxe, L. H. and Schmidt, E. M. (1953). *Trimitus parvus* Grassé (protozoa, mastigophora) from a garter snake *Thamnophis radix*. *Proc. Iowa Acad. Sci.* **60**, 754–758.

Schöppler, H. (1917). Ueber eine pemphigusartige Erkrankung bei *Lacerta agilis*, durch Gregarinen hervorgerufen. *Zbl. Bakt.* I, **79**, 27–29.

Setna, S. B. and Bana, R. E. (1935). *Eimeria flaviviridis* n. sp. from the gallbladder of *Hemidactylus flaviviridis*. *J. roy. micr. Soc.* Ser. III, **55**, 256–260.

Shortt, H. E. and Swaminath, C. S. (1931). Life history and morphology of *Trypanosoma phlebotomi* (Mackie, 1914). *Indian J. med. Res.* **19**, 541–564.

Steck, F. (1962). Pathogenese und klinisches Bild der Amoebendysenterie der Reptilien. *Acta Trop.* **19**, 318–354.

Tiegs, O. W. (1931). Note on the occurrence of *Sarcocystis* in muscle of python. *Parasitology* **23**, 412–414.

Wood, W. F. (1953). Some observations on the intestinal protozoa of Californian lizards. *J. Parasit.* **21**, 165–174.

Yakimoff, W. L. and Gousseff, F. F. (1934). *Isospora phisalix* n. sp. eine neue Schlangencoccidie. *Arch. Protistenk.* **81**, 547–550.

Yakimoff, W. L. and Gousseff, F. F. (1935a). Une coccidie de serpent. *Ann. Parasit. hum. comp.* **13**, 28–31.

Yakimoff, W. L. and Gousseff, F. F. (1935b). On the coccidia of shrews, grass snakes and lizards. *J. Roy. micr. Soc.* Ser. III, **55**, 170–173.

C. TURBELLARIA

A few representatives of this group, the Temnocephala, may occasionally be found on turtles. The Sub-order varies from other turbellarians by the presence of peculiar tentacles and adhesive organs. They are harmless ectocommensals which feed on the remains of their host's diet. Some parasitic Temnocephala occur on crustaceans and snails in tropical climates. They were discovered in Chile in 1840 and were at first thought to be leeches (Hyman, 1951). Those which live on turtles pass their whole developmental cycle on the same host. A detailed account of these turbellarians was given by Baer (1931) and Bresslau and Reisinger (1926). Cordero (1946) described a most interesting case in which the Temnocephala were, in turn, parasitized by plerocercoids.

The particular species observed on turtles is *Temnocephalus brevicornis* Monticelli (Fig. 313. 3). It has been found in the arm-pit and on the tail of *Hydromedusa tectifera* Cope, *H. maximiliani* Mikan, *H. platanensis* Gray, *Platemys radiolata* Mikan and *Mesoclemmys gibba* Schweigg.

Merten (1922) suspected *Temnocephalus brasiliensis* to live on turtles. He described the morphology of this species and that of a variation, *Temnocephalus brevicornis* Monticelli which he calls *var. intermedia*. It seems possible that neither species is entirely specific with regard to their host. Boettger (1957) saw *T. brevicornis* not only on turtles but on freshwater crustaceans as well.

REFERENCES

Baer, J. G. (1931). Étude monographique du groupe des Temnocephales. *Bull. biol.* **65**, 1–57.

Boettger, C. R. (1957). Stammesgeschichte und Verbreitung der Turbellariengruppe *Temnocephalida. Abh. Braunschw. wiss. Ges.* **9**, 26–35.

Bresslau, E. and Reisinger, E. (1926). *Temnocephalida. In* "Handbuch der Zoologie" (Kükenthal, ed.), Vol. 2, 294–308.

Cordero, E. H. (1946). *Ophiotaenia cohospes* n. sp. de la tortuga fluvial *Hydromedusa tectifera* Cope, una larva plerocercoide en el parenquima de *Temnocephala brevicornis* Mont., y su probable metamorfosis. *Comm. zool. mus. hist. nat. Montevideo* **2**, Nr. 34, 1–12.

Hyman, L. H. (1951). "The Invertebrates", Vol. II. McGraw-Hill, New York.

Merten, H. (1922). Ergebnisse einer zoologischen Forschungsreise in Brasilien 1913–14 von E. Bresslau. Neue Beiträge zur Anatomie von Temnocephala. *Zool. Jahrb. Anat.* **43**, 539–556.

D. TREMATODA

Monogenea

The trematodes (flat-worms with suckers) are among the commonest of parasites. Many of them are found in reptilians, most of them belonging to the Class Digenea which need one or several intermediate hosts to complete their life cycle. A few, however, are found among the Monogenea which need no intermediate host and the Aspidobothria which have very large suckers, subdivided by septa. Other genera of Monogenea found in reptiles are those of *Polystoma* and *Polystomoidella*.

Rudolphi (1819) was the first to describe finding a monogenetic trematode in a reptile. He found the worm in the oral cavity of *Emys orbicularis* L. and called it *Polystoma ocellatum*. It is now known as *Polystomoides ocellatum* (Stunkard, 1924; Paul, 1938). The genus was established by Stunkard (1924). It represents only reptilian parasites, among them *Polystomoides multifalx* St. and *P. oris* Paul (1938) from

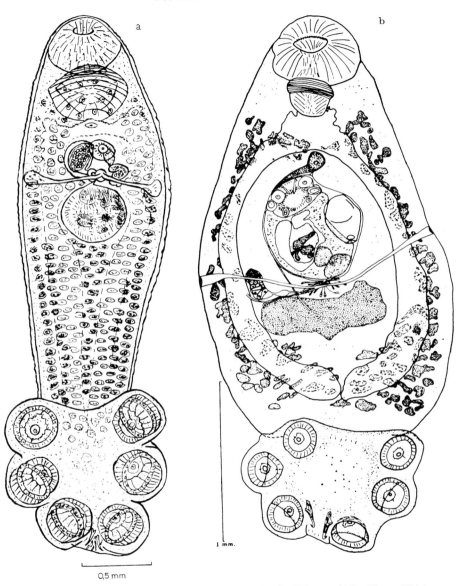

Fig. 306. (a) *Polystomoides oris* Paul. (From Paul.); (b) *Polystomoidella oblonga* Wright. (From Oglesby.)

the mouth of *Chrysemys picta* Schn. (Fig. 306a). Paul recorded trematodes in eighteen out of fifty-seven turtles, some harbouring up to five worms. Oglesby (1961) published a detailed study on *Polystomoidella oblonga* Wright from the urinary bladder of *Sternotherus odoratus* Latreille (Fig. 306b).

The urinary bladder is the commonest habitat of monogenetic trematodes both in amphibians and reptiles. They are less frequently seen in the nasal or oral cavities, in the oesophagus or on the carapace. Only one species, *Neopolystoma orbiculare* has been found in the lungs.

Sproston (1949) gives the following key to the genus, limited to species found on reptiles:

(1) Adhesive organ without hooks   *Neopolystoma*
    Adhesive organ with one or two pairs of hooks   2
(2) One pair of hooks   *Polystomoidella*
    Two pairs of hooks   *Polystomoides*

The three genera differ from the main genus *Polystoma*, mainly found in amphibians, by a shorter uterus which contains only one egg and the presence of only one testis.

Sproston (1949) lists the following species as occurring on reptilians:

Neopolystoma domitilae Price in the urinary bladder of *Pseudemys ornata* Gray;

N. rugosum Price in the nostrils of *Trionyx ferox* Schn.;

N. orbiculare Price in the urinary bladder of *Pseudemys scripta elegans* Wied and related species like *Chrysemys picta* Schn., *C. picta marginata* Agassiz, *Chelodina longicollis* Shaw, *Malaclemmys centrata* Latr. and in the lungs and the gut of *Trionyx ferox*;

N. chelodinae Price in the urinary bladder of *Chelodina longicollis* Shaw;

N. exhamatum Price in the urinary bladder of *Clemmys japonica* Temm. and Schl.;

N. palpebrae Strelkow in *Trionyx sinensis* Wiegmann (Bychowsky, 1957);

N. terrapenis Price in the urinary bladder of *Terrapene carolina triunguis* Ag.;

Polystomoidella oblonga (Wright) Price in the urinary bladder and on the carapace of *Kinosternon scorpioides integrum* Le Conte, other species of *Kinosternon*, *Sternotherus carinatus* Gray, other species of *Sternotherus* and *Chelydra serpentina* L.;

P. hassalli Price (? = *oblonga*) in the urinary bladder of *Kinosternon* spp. and *Chelydra serpentina* L.;

P. whartoni Price in the urinary bladder of *Kinosternon* spp.;

Polystomoides ocellatus (Rud.) Ozaki, in the mouth, pharynx and nostrils of *Emys orbicularis* L., *Chelone mydas* L., and *Caretta caretta* L.;

P. coronatus Price in the mouth and the nostrils of various *Pseudemys,*
Chrysemys, Graptemys, Malaclemmys and *Trionyx* species as well as
in *Chelydra serpentina* L., and *Terrapene carolina triunguis* Agassiz.;

P. oris Paul in the mouth of *Chrysemys picta* Schn.;

P. japonicus Ozaki in the mouth and the pharynx of *Clemmys
japonica* Temm. and Schl.;

P. megaovum Ozaki in the urinary bladder of *Geoemyda spengleri*
Gmelin.;

P. kachugae Fukui and Ogata in the mouth of *Ocadia sinensis* Gray;

P. ocadiae Fukui and Ogata in the mouth of *Ocadia sinensis* Gray;

P. multifalx (Stunkard) Ozaki in the mouth and the pharynx of
Pseudemys scripta elegans Wied.;

P. digitatum MacCallum in *Trionyx s. spinifera* Le Sueur and *Trionyx
ferox* Schn. (perhaps synonymous with *P. coronatus*);

P. opacum Stunkard in *Trionyx ferox* Schn. and *Graptemys geographica* Le Sueur (probably synonymous with *P. coronatus*).

Aspidobothria

Family Aspidogastridae

Differing from all other trematodes the Aspidogastridae are equipped
with a very large ventral adhesive organ subdivided by septa into 27–
144 single suckers. The parasites penetrate deeply into the body of the
host. They have been seen in fish, molluscs, crustaceans and also in
chelonians. They have no typical metamorphosis and do not usually
change their host, but if their host is devoured by another animal they
may survive and appear in an accidental host.

Dollfus (1958) investigated the Aspidogastridae, supplying a key
and a morphological description of the family. Nothing is known so
far about a possible pathogenic effect of these worms on their hosts.
The author lists the following species as having been found in reptilians:

Lophotaspis interiora Ward and Hopkins in the gut of *Macrochelys
temmincki* Holbrook (= *Macroclemmys temmincki* Troost?);

L. orientalis Faust and Tang in stomach and gut of *Trionyx sinensis*
Wiegman, China;

L. vallei Stossich in the oesophagus and the stomach of *Caretta
caretta* L. Eastern mediterranean; east coast of tropical America;

Multicotyle purvisi Dawes from *Siebenrockiella crassicollis* Gray,
Malaya (adhesive organ with 144 suckers);

Lissemysia indica Simha in the gut of *Lissemys punctata* Gray, India;

Cotylaspis cokeri Barker and Pearsons in the gut of *Graptemys
pseudogeographica* Gray, N. America;

C. lenoiri Poirier in the gut of *Cyclanorbis senegalenensis* Dum. and
Bibr. Senegal, and *Trionyx triunguis* Forsk. Nile;

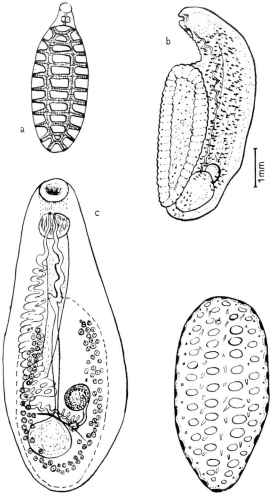

Fig. 307. a, *Cotylaspis cokeri* Barker and Pearsons; b, *Lophotaspis vallei* Stossich; c,
Lophotaspis orientalis Faust and Tang. ×15. On the right an adhesive disk. (From
Dollfus.)

C. sinensis Faust and Tang in the gut of *Trionyx sinensis* Wiegman,
China;

C. stunkardi Rumbold in the gut of *Chelydra serpentina* L. N. America.
Details of the parasites concerned are shown in the illustrations (Fig.

307). For the determination of species the original publication (Dollfus, 1958) should be consulted.

Digenetic Trematodes of the Intestinal Canal

About 200 different species of host-changing trematodes may be found, as mature worms in reptilians, mostly inhabiting the intestinal tract. The complete life cycle has only been worked out in a few species; the first intermediate host is, in most cases, a mollusc. The reptile usually becomes infected by feeding upon the second intermediate host. For the genus *Eustomos* mud snails (Lymnaeidae) serve as the first; dragonfly larvae as second intermediate hosts. In *Telorchis* the first host is again a snail of the genus *Physella*, while larval amphibians represent the second intermediate host.

Family Plagiorchidae

Many typical genera of this family, which makes up most of the digenetic trematodes occurring in reptilians, are found in this group:

Leptophallus. A genus particularly represented by L. *nigrovenosus* Bellingham frequently seen in the gut of snakes. First intermediate host lymnaeid snails, second host Amphibia (Fig. 308c);

Opisthioglyphe spp. parasitize snakes and chelonians. *O. ranae* Frölich (Fig. 309b) appears in snakes and amphibians. The snakes may become infected by feeding on the frogs;

Plagiorchis lives in chameleons, lizards and snakes. Example: *P. mentulatus* St. (Fig. 308a);

Astiotrema spp. which occur in snakes and chelonians, have been described by Mehra (1931b) (Fig. 308e);

Styphlodora. Dawes (1941b) found representatives of this genus in chelonians, snakes and varanids.

Rarer genera, occasionally seen in chelonians, are *Rhytidodes*; *Rhytodo-doides*; *Pachypsolus*; *Styphlotrema* and *Enodiotrema*. The original papers (Dawes, 1948; Yamaguti, 1958; Skrjabin, 1947) give details suitable for the determination of any of these species.

Renifer. Four species have been found in the gut of N. American snakes (Kagan, 1947). The Sub-family Reniferinae has been described by MacMullen and Talbot (1933);

Eustomos. *E. chelydrae* MacCallum (Fig. 310a) uses lymnaeid snails as first, dragonfly larvae as second intermediate host;

Zeugorchis spp. are frequently found in the stomach of snakes. Example: *Z. natricis* Holl and Allison (Fig. 310c);

Cercolecithos arrectus Molin parasitizes the gut of lizards;

Dasymetra spp., *Mediorina* spp. occur in snakes, *Tremiorchis* spp. in

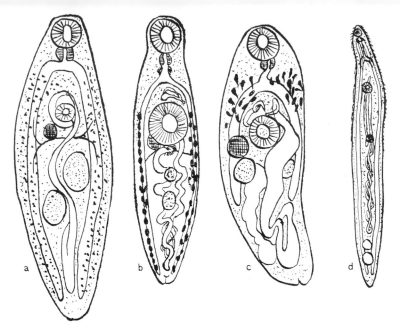

Fig. 308. Intestinal trematodes. I. a, *Plagiorchis mentulatus* Stossich; b, *Encyclometra caudata* Joyeux and Houdemer; c, *Leptophallus nigrovenosus* Bellingham; d, *Telorchis assula* Duj. (= *nematoides*) Mühling. (From Dawes.)

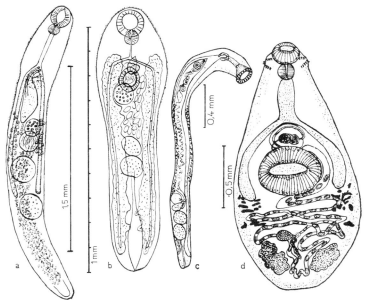

Fig. 309. Intestinal trematodes. II. a, *Astiotrema monticelli* Stossich. (After Dollfus.) b, *Opisthioglyphe ranae* Frölich (= *natricis* Dollfus); c, *Atrophocaecum indicum* Simha; d, *Singhiatrema singhia* Simha. (From Simha.)

Varanus; *Opisthogonimus interrogatus* Nicoll in snakes and *Microderma elinguis* Mehra in *Kachuga smithii* Gray.

Paralepoderma. The species *cloacicola* occurs in the common viper (*Vipera berus* L.). The first intermediate hosts are *Planorbis* snails. From them the parasite is transferred to frogs and toads but it can also accidentally appear in water beetles.

Spinometra. The genus was established by Mehra (1931a) for a parasite found on a turtle (*Spinometra kachugae* M.).

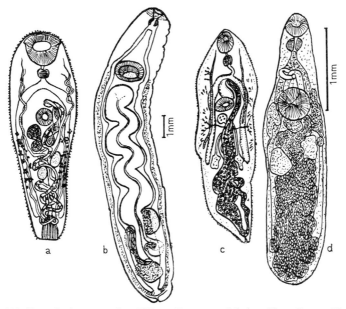

FIG. 310. Intestinal trematodes. III. a, *Eustomos chelydrae* Maccallum. × 32. (From Dawes.) b, *Odhneriotrema incommodum* Leidy. (From Dawes.) c, *Zeugorchis natricis* Holl and Allison. d, *Styphlodora compactum* Dawes. (From Dawes.)

Family Acanthostomatidae. Simha described *Atrophocaecum indicum* from Indian adders. Other Indian snakes were found infested by *Haplocaecum asymetricum* Simha (Fig. 309c). *Acanthostomum* occurs on crocodiles.

Family Allocreadidae. Only one species is known, *Crepidostomum cooperi* Hopkins from *Trionyx mutica* Webb.

Family Clinostomatidae. Several species of the genus *Odhneriotrema*; *O. microcephala* Travassos, and *O. incommodum* Leidy occur in crocodiles (Fig. 310b).

Family Cyathocotylidae. Simha describes *Gogata serpentum* v. *indicum* from the gut of several Indian snakes.

Family Dicrocoeliidae. *Brachycoelium salamandrae* Frölich, normally found in salamanders, occurs frequently in the slow-worm (*Anguis fragilis* L.). Simha described members of the genus *Paradistomoides* from lizards and chameleons.

Family Encyclometridae. *Encyclometra caudata* Joyeux and Baer, *E. natricis* Baylis and Cannon and *E. colubrimurorum* Rud. have been found in the gut of snakes, the latter species also in the oesophagus (Fig. 308b).

Family Echinostomidae. Species of *Singhiatrema* parasitize Indian snakes, *Paryphostomum* has been found in *Uromastix hardwicki* Gray.

Family Hemiuridae. Representatives of this family occur mainly in fish. The genera *Hemiurus* and *Lecithochirium* occur in chelonians, *Halipegus mehransis* Srivasta in the Indian snake *Ptyas mucosus* L.

Family Lecithodendriidae. Many species representing this family occur in lizards and chameleons, the latter may be parasitized by *Pleurogenoides gastroporus* Lühe and Travassos. Simha (1958) describes species of *Prosthodendrium* from Indian lizards as well as *Ganeo tigrinum* Mehra and Negi from Sinhalese chameleons. The genera *Orchidasma* and *Prosotocus* occur in lizards and chelonians; *Anchitrema sanguineum* Sansino and Looss also inhabits Sinhalese chameleons (Simha, 1958).

Family Microscaphidiidae. These are rarely seen parasites from marine turtles. Genera: *Polyangium, Octangium, Microscaphidium.*

Family Otobrephidae. These are parasites of Indian snakes.

Family Paramphistomidae. Chelonian parasites. Genera: *Parmaphistomum, Allostoma, Amphistoma, Stunkardia* (Bhalerao, 1931).

Family Pronocephalidae. Chelonian parasites. Genera: *Adenogaster, Pyelosomum, Diaschistorchis* (Rhode, 1962).

Family Proterodiplostomoidae. Simha (1958) found *Proalarioides tropidonotus* Vidyarthi in the gut of *Natrix piscator* Schn.

Family Telorchiidae. Odening (1960) reports *Telorchis assula* Duj. (= *T. ercolani* Mont.) as fairly common in *Natrix natrix* L. (Fig. 308d). Other representatives of this genus occur in snakes and chelonians. The life cycle of *Telorchis medius* Stunkard has been described. It begins with *Physella* snails. The infection is transmitted to a second host, an amphibian larva through which it reaches the final host, a snake or a turtle.

Digenetic Trematodes in the Gall Bladder, the Peritoneal Cavity, the Uterus and the Kidneys

Trematodes which have gained access to other organs of the host than the intestinal canal are a far greater menace to the health of the host than the former. Those found in the gall bladder are, in most cases, close relations of the intestinal species. Among the Plagiorchidae the genera *Allopharynx* and *Xenopharynx* are specialized in this direction (Simha, 1958) and inhabit the gall bladder of snakes. The same habitat is occupied by the Lecithodendriidae: *Mehraorchis chamaeleonis* Simha and *Paradistomum mutabile* Nicoll. In the gall bladder of lizards we find *Paradistomoides mutabile* Nicoll (Dicrocoeliidae).

The peritoneal cavity is not normally the seat of mature worms but is sometimes invaded by larval stages. The tortoise *Kachuga kachuga* Gray has been found peritoneally infected by *Isoparorchis hypselibagri* Billet (Family Sclerodistomatidae) (Simha, 1958).

Two plagiorchids, *Leptophyllum tamiamensis* McIntosh and *Zeugorchis aequatus* Stafford have been found in the uterus of snakes.

Even the kidney has, on occasion, been found invaded by mature worms. Snakes were found so infected by the plagiorchids *Paurophyllum simplexus* Byrd, Parker and Reiber and *P. megametricus* Byrd, Parker and Reiber (1940).

Digenetic Trematodes in the Lungs

The pulmonary parasites, very common in reptilians, deserve special attention. *Macrodera longicollis* Lühe, a common pulmonary parasite of snakes, may serve as an example (Fig. 311a). It is easily recognized by the club-shaped anterior end. In chelonians the commonest lung trematode is *Heronimus chelydrae* MacCallum, particularly found in *Chelydra serpentina* L. and *Chrysemys picta bellii* Gray (Fig. 311e). The first intermediate hosts are planorbid snails: *Gyraulus parvus* Say, physids (*Physa gyrini* Say), *Physa sayii* Tappan or *Valvata tricarinata* Say. Ulmer and Sommer (1957) succeeded in carrying out experimental infections. A sporocyst of this type of parasite is shown in Fig. 311f.

Several Plagiorchidae also occur in reptilian lungs. Apart from several species of *Styphlodora* we may find *Pneumatophilus variabilis* Leidy; *Caudorchis eurineus* Talbot as well as *Lechriorchis primus* Stafford; and *L. tygarti* Talbot. The latter four species live as mature worms in the lungs of several species of *Thamnophis* and *Natrix*. Talbot (1933) determined *Physella* as first, *Rana* tadpoles as second intermediate hosts.

Digenetic Trematodes of Liver and Circulatory System

Systematically there is close similarity between the hepatic and the circulatory trematodes. They are therefore treated together. The species coming under this heading all belong to the genus *Spirorchis*. Some types are highly specialized for a life in the circulatory system.

Simha (1958) found *Hepatohaematrema hepaticum* S. in the liver of *Kachuga kachuga* Gray. Martin and Bamberger (1952) gave a detailed description of trematodes found in reptilian blood vessels. They found *Haemoxenicon stunkardi* and *H. chelonenecon* in the veins of *Chelonia*

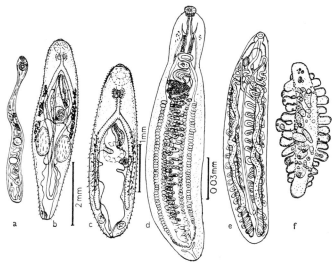

FIG. 311. Pulmonary and cardiac trematodes. a, *Macrodera longicollis* Lühe. (From Dawes.) b, *Lechriorchis primus* Stafford. (From Talbot.) c, *Caudorchis eurineus* Talbot. d, *Haemoxenicon chelonenecon* Martin and Bamberger. e, *Heronimus chelydrae* Maccallum. × 4. (After Stunkard.) f, 24 days old sporocyst of the same species. (After Ulmer and Sommer.)

mydas L. and described the species in detail. The worms have a predilection for the mesenteric veins which they sometimes block altogether. In the blood of marine turtles like *Chelone mydas* L. we may find *Learedius orientalis* Mehra, *L. learedi* Price and *L. similis* Price. *Amphiorchis amphiorchis* Price and *Monticellius indicus* Mehra also occur in marine turtles. Related species are: *Amphiorchis lateralis* Oguro from *Eretmochelys imbricata* L., the hawksbill turtle and *Carettacola bipora* Manter and Larson from *Caretta caretta* L., the loggerhead turtle. For a detailed description of these and the following trematodes the original papers must be consulted (see Yamaguti, 1958).

Both the circulatory and the cardiac trematodes have so far only been found in chelonians. Among them should be mentioned *Neospirorchis pricei* Manter and Larson from *Caretta caretta* L. and *Haplotrema synorchis* Luhmann as well as *H. constrictum* Leared from the same host.

Only one trematode, *Haplotrema polesianum* Ejsmont, has so far been found in the heart of the European turtle *Emys orbicularis* L.

Cercariae

Reptiles may occasionally carry encysted larval stages of digenetic trematodes, but they do not, in these cases, represent the natural second intermediate hosts; they only function as means of transport. Odening (1916) found large numbers of encapsulated cercariae of *Neodiplostomulum* sp. Nr. 2 Odening (? = *N. spathoides*) in the fatty tissue of a grass snake (*Natrix natrix* L.) and he compares these with similar types found in the Volga delta. The proper secondary intermediate hosts would in this case have been frogs, the final hosts birds of prey (Fig. 312).

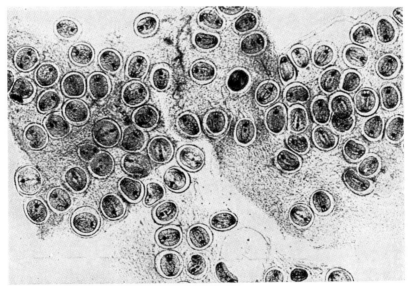

FIG. 312. *Neodiplostomulum* sp. No. 2 Odening (? = *spathoides* Dubois) from the fat body of a grass snake. Approx. × 25. (Photo.: Bockhardt. From Odening, 1961.)

The same author deals also with the appearance of the mesocercaria *Alaria alata* Göze in snakes. Here, too, the snakes serve only as secondary or transport intermediary hosts. The cercariae were found both in the grass snake (*Natrix natrix* L.) and the common viper (*Vipera berus* L.). The first intermediate hosts are, in this case, planorbid snails, the second ranid frogs and *Pelobates fuscus* Laur. The final host of *Alaria alata* is a carnivorous mammal. Small mammals may also on occasion function as secondary transport hosts for these cercariae.

REFERENCES

Bhalerao, G. D. (1931). Two new trematodes from reptiles: *Paryphostomum indicum* n. sp. and *Stunkardia dilymphosa* n. gen. n. sp. *Parasitology* **32**, 99–108.

Bychowsky, B. E. (1957). "Monogenetic Trematodes, their Systematics and Phylogeny." (W. J. Hargis, jr., ed.). Washington.

Byrd, E. E. (1936). A new trematode parasite from the mud turtle *Kinosternon subrubrum* Gray. *J. Pa: asit.* **22**, 413, 415.

Byrd, E. E., Parker, M. V. and Reiber, R. J. (1940). A new genus and two new species of digenetic trematodes with a discussion of the systematics of these and certain related forms. *J. Parasit.* **26**, 111–122.

Caballero, R. (1960). Estudio de trematodes digeneos de algunas tortugas comestibles de Mexico. Thesis Univ. Nac., Mexico.

Crandell, R. B. (1960). The life history and affinities of the turtle lung fluke *Heronimus chelydrae* MacCallum. *J. Parasit.* **46**, 289–307.

Dawes, B. (1941a). On *Multicotyle purvisi* n. g. n. sp., an Aspidogastrid trematode from the river turtle *Siebenrockiella crassicollis* in Malaya. *Parasitology* **33**, 300–305.

Dawes, B. (1941b). On *Styphlodora elegans* n. sp. and *Styphlodora compactum* n. sp. trematode parasites of *Python reticulatus* in Malaya, with a key to the species of the genus *Styphlodora* Looss 1889. *Parasitology* **33**, 445–458.

Dawes, B. (1956). "The Trematoda. With special reference to British and other European forms." Cambridge University Press.

Dollfus, R. P. (1958). Cours d'Helminthologie (1). I. Trematodes. Sousclasse *Aspidogastraea*. *Ann. Parasit. hum. comp.* **33**, 305–395.

Holl, F. J. and Allison, L. N. (1933). *Zeugorchis natricis* n. sp., a trematode from the water snake. *J. Parasit.* **21**, 274–276.

Kagan, F. G. (1947). A new species of *Renifer* (Trematoda) from the King Snake *Lampropeltis getulus*, with an emendation of the genus *Renifer* Pratt 1903. *J. Parasit.* **33**, 427–432.

Luhmann, M. (1933). Two new trematodes from the loggerhead turtle (*Caretta caretta*). *J. Parasit.* **21**, 274–276.

Martin, W. E. and Bamberger, J. W. (1952). New blood flukes (*Trematoda: Spirorchidae*) from the marine turtle *Chelonia mydas* L. *J. Parasit.* **38**, 105–110.

McIntosh, A. (1933). *Odhneriotrema incommodum* Leidy 1856, a trematode from the mouth of *Alligator mississippiensis* Daud. *J. Parasit.* **21**, 53–55.

McMullen, D. B. (1932). The life cycle of the turtle trematode *Cercorchis medius*. *J. Parasit.* **20**, 248–250.

McMullen, D. B. (1933). The life cycle and a discussion of the systematics of the turtle trematode, *Eustomos chelydrae*. *J. Parasit.* **21**, 52–53.

Mehra, H. R. (1931a). A new genus (*Spinometra*) of the Family Lepodermatidae Odhner (Trematoda) from a tortoise, with a systematic discussion and classification of the Family. *Parasitology* **23**, 157–178.

Mehra, H. R. (1938b). On two new species of the genus *Astiotrema* Loss belonging to the family Lepodermat dae Odhner. *Parasitology* **23**, 179–190.

Mehra, H. R. (1931c). On a new Trematode, *Microderma elinguis* n. g., n. sp. *Parasitology* **23**, 191–195.

Odening, K. (1960a). Zur Kenntnis einiger Trematoden aus Schlangen. *Zool. Anz.* **165**, 337–348.

Odening, K. (1960b). Studien an Trematoden aus Schlangen, Vögeln und Säugetieren. *Monat. dtsch. Akad. Wiss. Bln.* **2**, 438–445.

Odening, K. (1961a). Weitere Mittelungen über Trematodenlarven vom Typ *Neodiplostomulum* aus einheimischen *Natrix natrix* L. sowie über erste Versuche zur Erforschung der Biologie dieser Larven. *Ibid.* **3**, 59–69.

Odening, K. (1961b). Zur Parasitenfauna europäischer Schlangen, unter besonderer Berücksichtigung ihrer Rolle im Zyklus des Erregers der Alariose. *Biol. Beitr.* **1**, 172–136.

Oglesby, L. C. (1961). Ovoviviparity in the monogenetic Trematode *Polystomoidella oblonga*. *J. Parasit.* **47**, 237–243.

Paul, A. A. (1938). Life history studies of N. American freshwater Polystomes. *J. Parasit.* **24**, 469–510.

Rhode, K. (1962). A new Trematode, *Diaschistorchis multitesticularis* sp. n. from a Malayan tortoise, *Hieremys annandalei* Boulenger. *J. Parasit.* **48**, 296–297.

Rudolphi, C. A. (1819). "Entozoorum Synopsis." Berlin.

Schewtschenko, N. N. and Barabaschowa, V. N. (1958). Helminth fauna of *Lacerta agilis* and *Vipera berus* L. in the Charkow area. *Izd. Akad. Nauk. SSSR.*, Festschr. Skrjabin 389–394.

Siddiqui, W. A. (1958). On a new Trematode, *Astiotrema geomydia* (Fam. Plagiorchidae) from an Indian tortoise. *Z. Parasitenk.* **18**, 219–222.

Simha, S. S. (1958). Studies on the Trematode parasites of reptiles found in Hyderabad State, *Z. Parasitenk.* **18**, 161–218.

Simha, S. S. (1960). Observations on *Anchitrema sanguineum* Sansino 1894, Looss 1988. *J. biol. Sci.* **3**, 46–47.

Skrjabin, K. J. (1947). "Trematody shiwotnych i tscheloweka." Moscow.

Sproston, N. G. (1949). A synopsis of the Monogenetic Trematodes. *Trans. zool. Soc. Lond.* **25**, 185–600.

Stunkard, H. W. (1924). On some trematodes from Florida turtles. *Trans. Amer. micr. Soc.* **43**, 97–110.

Talbot, S. B. (1933). Life history studies on trematodes of the Sub-family Reniferinae. *Parasitology* **25**, 518–545.

Thapar, G. S. (1933). On a new Trematode of the genus *Astiotrema*, Looss 1900, from the intestine of a tortoise. *Chitra indica*. *J. Helminth.* **11**, 87–94.

Waitz, J. A. (1961). Parasites of Idaho reptiles. *J. Parasit.* **47**, 51.

Yamaguti, S. (1958). "Systema Helminthum", Vol. I. Interscience, London, New York.

E. TAPEWORMS (CESTOIDEA)

Sub-class Cestodes

Both the larvae and the mature stages of these worms may be encountered in reptilians, either in the intestine or in the peritoneal cavity. The reptiles become infected by feeding on other animals parasitized by larval cestodes. If the infestation is heavy, the reptiles may become weakened. Particularly large tapeworms may also be pathogenic simply because of their size.

The following cestodes have recently been described from reptiles from the Rhodesias (Mettrick, 1963):

Ophiotaenia ophiodes: From *Causus rhombeatus.*
Ophiotaenia punica: From *Causus rhombeatus.*
Ophiotaenia theileri: From *Causus rhombeatus.*
Ophiotaenia nigricollis sp. n.: From *Naja nigricollis crawshayi* Gthr.
Diphyllobothriidae:
Bothridium pithonis: From *Python sebae* var. *minus.*
Duthiersia fimbriata: From *Varanus niloticus.*
Anoplocephalidae:
Megacapsula leiperi: From *Pachydactylus bibroni.*
the latter is probably identical with *Oochoristica agamae* Baylis 1919.

Order Proteocephaloidea

Members of the genera *Acanthotaenia* and *Ophiotaenia* are commonly seen in the reptilian gut. The former genus is mostly found in lizards, the latter in snakes and chelonians.

Acanthotaenia, a genus with at least twelve species, is distinguished by the presence of fine spines on the scolex. These spines are missing in the allied genus *Ophiotaenia* (fifty species) (Figs. 313, 316a). Many of the species described are of uncertain validity and frequent synonymity cannot be excluded. Among the more commonly seen species are *Ophiotaenia perspicua* La Rue, *O. zschokkei* Rudin and *O. agkistrodontis* Harwood, Less frequently seen are *Crepidobothrium gerrardii* Baird which occurs in snakes and the doubtful species *Palaia varani* Shipley from *Varanus indicus* Daud.

The first intermediate host of all these Proteocephaloidea is a copepode which takes up cestode eggs with its food. The larva develops in the crustacean and changes into the procercoid. Although neither snakes nor lizards feed on copepodes the procercoid somehow gains access to these reptiles, perhaps by way of making use of other intermediate hosts like amphibian larvae or fish. *Ophiotaenia perspicua* La Rue is one of the few species where the life cycle has been experimentally determined.

Order Trypanorhyncha

Most of the members of this Order parasitize marine selachians (sharks and rays). It is therefore remarkable that they also occur in reptiles. The Trypanorhyncha are recognized by their long cephalic tentacles which are armed with hooks (Fig. 314).

Otobothrium cysticum Mayer has been found in the gut of the marine turtle *Chelonia mydas* L. The larva of the worm lives in marine fish which serve as food to the turtle which also serves as host to another cestode, *Tentacularia coryphaenae* Bosc. Larvae of this species have been discovered in fish of the genus *Coryphaena*.

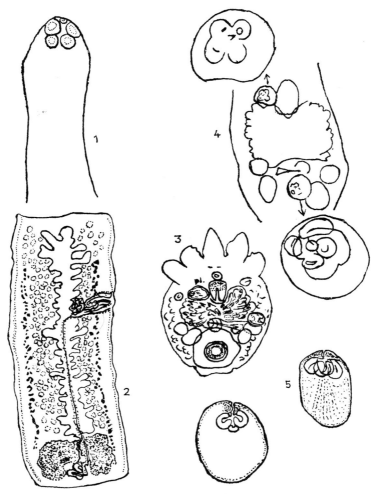

Fig. 313. 1 and 2. *Ophiotaenia cohospes* Cordero (1946). 3 and 4. *Temnocephala brevicornis* Monticelli. 5. Larval stages. (From Cordero, 1946.)

We may further note the appearance of Trypanorhyncha in marine snakes, even in crocodiles, and, in one case, in the peritoneal cavity of the horned viper *Aspis cerastes* L. whose habitat, the Sahara, is far distant from the sea (Dollfus, 1957) (Fig. 314).

Order Cyclophyllidea

Apart from the genus *Ophiotaenia*, reptilian cestodes are represented by another group, the *Oochoristica*. Wardle and McLeod (1952) dis-

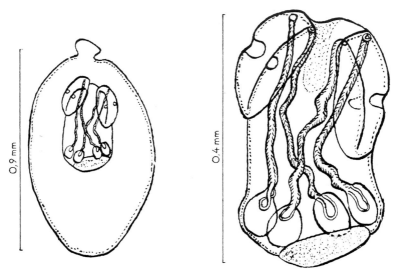

FIG. 314. Plerocercoid of *Otobothrium* (?). (After Dollfus.)

tinguish twenty-two species in lizards, snakes and chelonians. Commonly seen are, for instance, *Oochoristica bivitellolobata* Loewen (Fig. 316b), *O. parvovaria* Steelman (Fig. 316c), *O. americana* Harwood, *O. anniellae* Stunkard and Lynch and *O. whitentoni* Steelman (Fig. 316d). All these are worms of moderate length, their proglottids are longer than wide. Their life cycle is fairly well known. Ticks function as first intermediate hosts harbouring the tapeworm larva, the cysticercus.

The only species of the related genus *Nematotaenia*, so commonly seen in amphibians, which occurs in reptiles is *Nematotaenia tarentolae* Lopez-Neyra found in geckos (Fig. 315).

Ophiovalipora houdemeri Hsü occurs in *Elaphe carinata*. The intermediate host is thought to be an insect. The life cycle of *Pancerina varani* Stossich is as yet unknown.

Cestodes of the related genus *Joyeuxella* pass their larval stage in lizards. A coprophagous insect, probably a fly, serves as intermediate host. The final hosts are mammals which become infected by feeding on reptiles. *Joyeuxella pasqualii* Diamare is a tapeworm of dog, wolf or cat, *J. echinorhynchoides* Sonsino matures in the fox or the dog.

Order Pseudophyllida

Only a few members of this Order mature in reptiles, where their larvae are, however, frequently seen.

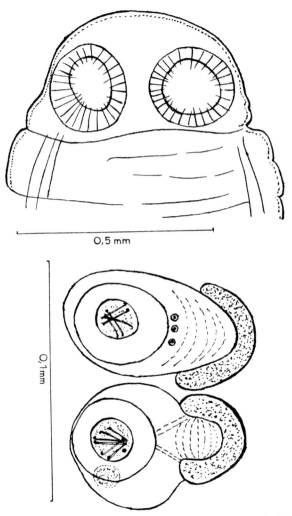

FIG. 315. Above: *Oochoristica rostellata* Zschokke var. *agamicola* Dollfus. Below: *Nematotaenia tarentolae* Lopez-Neyra. Two egg capsules with parauterine organs. (From Dollfus.)

The mature worm of *Spirometra serpentis* Yamaguti may be found in *Naja naja atra* Cantor. *Python molurus* L. may be infested by

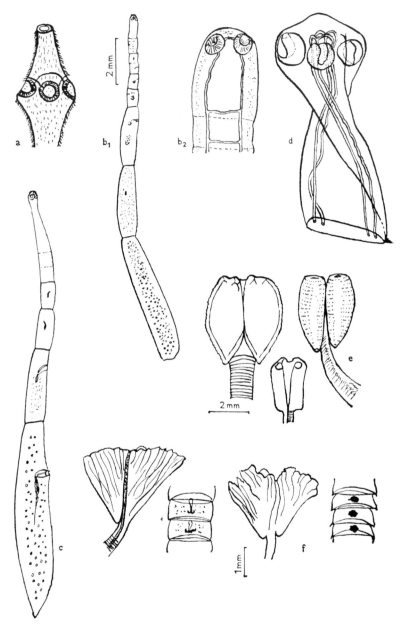

FIG. 316. Cestodes from reptiles. (From Wardle and MacLeod.) a, *Acanthotaenia shipleyi* Linstow. Scolex. (After Southwell.) b, *Oochoristica bivitellolobata* Loewen. c, *Oochoristica parvovaria* Steelman. d, *Oochoristica whitentoni* Steelman. e, *Bothridium pithonis* Blainville. (From Southwell and Joyeux, Du Noyer and Baer, 1931.) f, *Duthiersia expansa* Perrier. (From Woodland.)

Bothridium pithonis Blainville and *Varanus* species by *Duthiersia expansa* Perrier and *D. fimbriata* Diesing. A more rarely seen species is *Ancistrocephalus imbricatus* Diesing, a triaenophorid which occurs in the marine turtle *Thalassochelys caretta* L. These worms, too, are of medium size with oblong proglottids (*Spirometra*) or with a club-shaped (*Bothridium*) or lobed scolex (Fig. 316e, f). Small crustaceans like *Cyclops* are the first intermediate hosts. They pick up the cestode eggs from the bottom and then act as hosts to the larval procercoids. It is as yet not known whether direct transmission takes place from the copepode to the reptile or whether a second intermediate host is required.

Numerous Pseudophyllidea have been reported from reptiles. Larval stages of *Spirometra erinacei* Faust, Campbell and Kellogg have been seen in snakes and lizards. The first intermediate host is again a *Cyclops*, final hosts are E. Asian dogs and foxes. Other sparganids may occur in frogs and may be transferred to humans when these frogs are used to cure eye diseases, a method said to have been popular in E. Asia. Similar sparganids, whose final hosts are carnivorous cats, have been found in crocodiles. The larva of *Diphyllobothrium reptans* Diesing, which occurs in snakes, has been described as "*Spirometra reptans* Meggit". The final hosts are dogs. Schreitmüller and Lederer (1930) found in snakes another sparganid, *Plerocercoides panceri* Polonio (= *Ligula panceri* Polonio). The mature worm is again found in carnivorous cats. Differentiation between these species is difficult and the systematics of the group consequently as yet unsatisfactory.

REFERENCES

Beddard, P. E. (1913). On some species of *Ichthyotaenia* and *Ophiotaenia* from Ophidia. *Proc. zool. Soc. Lond.* **1913**, 153–168.

Cordero, E. H. (1946). *Ophiotaenia cohospes* n. sp. de la tortuga fluvial *Hydromedusa tectifera* Cope, una larva plerocercoide en el perenquina de *Temnocephala brevicornis* Mont., y su probable metamorfosis. *Comm. Zool. Mus. Hist. Nat. Montevideo* II, **34**, 1–12.

Dollfus, R. P. (1957). Présence accidentelle d'une larve de Cestode tetrarhynque chez un Ophidien terrestre d'Algérie. *Ann. Inst. Pasteur, Algérie* **35**, 70–72.

Harwood, P. D. (1933). The helminths parasitic in a water moccasin (snake) with a discussion of the character of the Proteocephalidae. *Parasitology* **25**, 130–142.

Hyman, L. H. (1951). "The Invertebrates", Vol. II. McGraw-Hill, New York.

Meggitt, F. J. (1933). On some tape worms from the bull snake (*Pituophis sayi*) with remarks on the species of the genus *Oochoristica* (*Cestoda*). *J. Parasit.* **20**, 181–189.

Mettrick, D. F. (1963). Some cestodes of reptiles and amphibians from the Rhodesias. *Proc. zool. Soc. Lond.* **141**, 239–250.

Mueller, J. P. (1951). Spargana from the Florida alligator. *J. Parasit.* **37**, 317–318.

Schreitmüller, W. and Lederer, G. (1930). "Krankheitserscheinungen an Fischen Reptilien und Lurchen." Wenzel, Berlin.
Southwell, T. (1928). Cestodes of the Order *Pseudophyllidea* recorded from India and Ceylon. *Amer. J. trop. Med.* **22**, 419–448.
Waitz, J. A. (1961). Parasites of Idaho reptiles. *J. Parasit.* **47**, 51.
Wardle, R. A. and McLeod, J. A. (1952). "The Zoology of Tape Worms." University of Minnesota Press, Minneapolis, U.S.A.

F. Acanthocephala

The Reptilia serve mainly as temporary or occasional hosts to these worms whose proboscis is armed with rows of barbed hooks. Of mature worms only one genus, *Neoechinorhynchus*, is sometimes seen in chelonians. Following upon the original description of one species of this genus (*N. emydis* Leidy) by Lincicome (1948), Cable and Hopp (1954) suggested that this description had probably been based on more than one species. The chelonian Acanthocephala are, in their view, very species-specific. They determined the further species *Neoechinorhynchus pseudemydis* and *N. chrysemydis*. There are further *N. emyditoides* Fisher and *N. stunkardi* Cable and Fisher (1961), the latter from *Graptemys pseudogeographica* Gray. Snails serve as primary intermediate hosts to all these species. The related species *N. rutili* Müller, a widely distributed parasite of fish, may occasionally be found in the stomach of turtles (Sprehn, 1959) (Fig. 317). The intermediate hosts are in this case *Sialis* larvae and Ostracodes (Finland).

Acanthocephalus anthuris Duj. (Fig. 318), commonly seen in amphibians, may also attack chelonians.

Acanthocephalus ranae Schrank, so commonly seen in frogs and toads, may be transferred to grass snakes (*Natrix natrix* L.) which infect themselves by feeding on the frogs. It is unlikely that they should feed on the intermediate hosts *Asellus aquaticus* L.

Snakes may serve as temporary hosts to species of the genera *Oligacanthorhynchus* and *Centrorhynchus*. The final hosts are in the main birds.

Frogs, lizards and adders function as intermediate hosts to *Centrorhynchus aluconis* Müller whose final hosts are ducks. *C. areolatus* Rud. and *C. lancea* Westrumb occur temporarily in *Coluber viridiaeneus;* the final hosts are birds of prey, intermediate hosts terrestrial insect larvae. Early stages of *C. lesiniformis* Molin and *C. leptorhynchus* Meyer have been found in *Natrix natrix* L. The first intermediate hosts of *C. cinctus* Rud. are terrestrial insects; further hosts amphibians and snakes, and final hosts birds of prey.

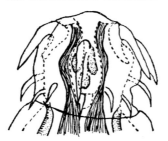

FIG. 317. *Neoechinorhynchus rutili* Müller. An occasional parasite in the stomach of *Emys orbicularis* L. Anterior extremity. (From Sprehn.)

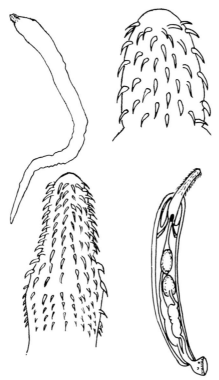

FIG. 318. Above: *Acanthocephalus ranae* Schrank, an occasional parasite of the grass snake. Left, the whole worm. × 4. Right, Anterior extremity. × 72. Below: *Acanthocephalus anthuris* Duj. × 72 and × 16. (From Lühe.)

The encysted juvenile forms of *C. buteonis* Schrank, a parasite of owls, have been found in lizards and snakes. These may also harbour *C. picae* Rud.

Rarer Acanthocephalus species, mentioned by Petrotschenko (1956/8) are: *Polyacanthorhynchus macrorhynchus* Baylis, a parasite of crocodiles, birds and fish and *Sphaerechinorhynchus rotundocapitatus* Johnston, which occurs in the Australian *Pseudechis porphyriacus* Shaw.

It seems, on the whole, as if reptilians infect themselves with Acanthocephala less through feeding on the first, but far more through ingesting second intermediary hosts, in particular Amphibia.

REFERENCES

Andruschko, A. M. and Markow, G. S. (1958). The helminth fauna of reptiles in the Kysil-Kum desert. *Isdt. Akad. Nauk. SSSR.* Festschr. Skrjabin, 32–37.
Cable, R. M. and Hopp, W. B. (1954). Acanthocephalan parasites of the genus *Neoechinorhynchus* in N. American turtles, with the description of two new species. *J. Parasit.* **40**, 674–680.
Cable, R. M. and Fisher, F. M. (1961). A fifth species of *Neoechinorhynchus* (Acanthocephala) in turtles. *J. Parasit.* **47**, 666–668.
Fisher, F. M. jr. (1960). On Acanthocephala of turtles, with the description of *Neoechinorhynchus emyditoides* n. sp. *J. Parasit.* **46**, 257–266.
Lincicome, D. R. (1948). Observations on *Neoechinorhynchus emydis* Leidy an acanthocephalan parasite of turtles. *J. Parasit.* **24**, 51–54.
Meyer, A. (1933). Acanthocephala. *In* Brohmer "Die Tierwelt Mitteleuropas" (Ehrmann and Ulmer, eds.). Quelle and Meyer, Leipzig.
Petrotschenko, V. J. (1956/8). "Akantocefaly domashnich i dikich shivotnych." (In Russian.) Moscow.
Sprehn, C. (1959). Acanthocephala. *In* "Die Tierwelt Mitteleuropas." (Supplement to Brohmer *et al.*). Quelle and Meyer, Leipzig.

G. NEMATODA

Nematodes are commonly seen in reptiles. They occur in the most varied organs, particularly in the intestine and the lungs. Their presence is the more serious to the host the more numerous the worms are, and this is particularly true in respect of the filaria inhabiting the bloodstream, where they can cause thrombosis and oedema. Single nematodes are rarely harmful, but may be dangerous to juvenile animals.

There is hardly a "pet" more widely distributed and more misunderstood than *Testudo graeca* L. the "European" or "Greek" tortoise which, in most cases, does not come from either Europe or Greece but from N. Africa. Those who keep these unfortunate reptiles in countries mostly much too cold for their comfort are sometimes alarmed to see that their pets are infested by intestinal worms. They may well be alarmed, for according to a recent investigation carried out by Shad (1963) Greek tortoises kept in his laboratory were found infected by eight different species of oxyurid worms. The account he gives of these worms is worth quoting. In ten female tortoises (weight and age are not given) he found the following species of *Tachygonetria:*

Species	No. of worms in 10 ♀ tortoises	Numbers of tortoises affected
1. *T. dentata*	7 138	10
2. *T. macrolaimus*	3 480	10
3. *T. conica*	1 942	10
4. *T. microstoma*	718	10
5. *T. robusta*	300	10
6. *T. stylosa*	723	7
7. *T. uncinata*	457	9
8. *T. numidica*	196	6

In other words, nearly half the tortoises were hosts to six different oxyurid species. They were all found in the colon from the ileo-colic juncture on down to the cloaca, but the distribution of the various species within the colon varied greatly. The author ascribes this "Niche diversification" to food or environmental preferences among the worms.

The following catalogue of nematodes parasitizing Reptilia is mainly based on the systematic papers of Yorke and Maplestone (1926), Chitwood and Chitwood (1950) and Skrjabin (1960).

Nematodes of the Intestinal Canal

Almost 500 different species of nematodes have been described from reptiles. Most of them inhabit the small intestine, some the colon and a few the stomach and the oesophagus.

(a) Ascaroidea

Ascarids are, as elsewhere, common intestinal parasites of reptiles, but we have no accounts so far of migrations within the host analogous to these occurring in mammals. Ash and Beaver (1962) investigated the occurrence of the ascarid *Ophidascaris labiatopapillosa* Walton and its life cycle. They discovered the larval stage of this parasite in the amphibium *Amphiuma tridactylum* Cuv. and in various frogs like *Rana pipiens* Gmel. and *Rana clamitans* Daud. The larvae were found either free or encysted in the liver or the mesenterium. The adult worm occurs in a variety of snakes of the genus *Natrix, Coluber, Lampropeltis* and *Heterodon*.

The following genera are more commonly encountered in reptiles:

Ascaris: One species only pathogenic for reptiles: *A. cephaloptera* Rud.

Hexametra: Ten intestinal parasites have been described from chameleons and from lizards (Fig. 319a).

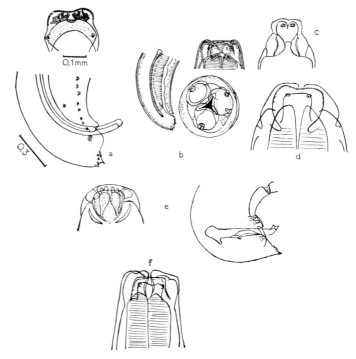

FIG. 319. Nematodes from the intestine of reptiles. *Ascaroidea, Anisakoidea.* a, *Hexametra sewelli* Baylis and Daubney. Anterior and posterior extremity. b, *Polydelphis dalmatina* Kreis. c, *Trispiculascaris trispiculascaris* Travassos, anterior extremity. (After Skrjabin from Yorke and Maplestone.) d, *Ophidascaris filaria* Baylis, anterior extremity. × 80. (From Yorke and Maplestone.) e, *Dujardinascaris helicina* Baylis. Anterior and posterior extremity. × 67. (After Baylis from Yorke and Maplestone.) f, *Angusticaecum holopterum* Baylis, anterior extremity. × 42. (From Yorke and Maplestone.)

Ophidascaris: More than twenty intestinal forms, mostly slender forms of medium size are known from snake and lizards. Genotype *O. filaria* Baylis (Fig. 319d).

The following species of *Ophidascaris* were listed by Baylis (1921):

Ophidascaris filaria Duj. 1845: From *Python molurus, Python reticulatus, Python sebae* and *Python spilotes*. It was also found in *Varanus* species in Zanzibar.

Ophidascaris radiosa Schneider 1866: From *Bitis gabonica.*

Ophidascaris obconica Baird 1860: From *Helicops angulatus* (Brazil).

Ophidascaris mombasica sp. nov.: From *Psammophis subtaeniatus* (Mombasa).

Ophidascaris gestri Parona 1890: From *Tropidonotus piscator* (*T. quincunciatus*).

Ophidascaris papillifera v. Linst: Undetermined snakes from the Bismarck archipelago.

Ophidascaris solitaria v. Linst.: From *Dipsadomorphus dendrophilus* (Siam).

Ophidascaris naiae Gedoelst 1916: From *Naja nigricollis* (Belgian Congo).

Ophidascaris intorta Gedoelst 1916: From *Bitis* spp. (Belgian Congo).

Polydelphis: Skrjabin described nine species, slender and of medium size, from snakes (Fig. 319b).

Baylis (loc. cit.) lists the following species of *Polydelphis*:

Polydelphis anoura Duj. 1845: From *Python molurus, Python sebae, Bitis arietans, Drymobius bifossatus* (= *Coluber lichtensteini*), *Coluber corais, Zamenis constrictor.*

Polydelphis attenuata Molin 1858: From *Python molurus, P. sebae, P. reticulatus, Bitis arietans.*

Polydelphis oculata v. Linst. 1899: From *Python reticulatus, P. sebae.*

Polydelphis quadricornis Wedl 1862: From *Naja haje, N. nigricollis, Bitis arietans, Pseudaspis cana, Crotalus* spp.

Polydelphis boddaerti Baird 1860: From *Drymobius boddaerti* (West Indies).

Polydelphis hexametra Gedoelst 1916: From *Chamaeleo dilepis* (Belgian Congo).

Polydelphis waterstoni sp. nov.: From *Zamenis gemonensis* var. *caspius* (Macedonia).

One of us (E. E.) recently found an undetermined species of *Polydelphis* in the sublingual pouch of a *Chamaeleo melleri* from Tanganyika.

Trispiculascaris: *Tr. trispiculascaris* Travassos inhabits the gut of crocodiles. It is the only species of the genus (Fig. 319c).

Other ascarid worms are listed by Baylis (loc. cit.) as occurring in crocodiles as follows:

Dujardinascaris helicina Baylis: From *Crocodilus niloticus* and other crocodile spp.

Typhlophorus lamellaris v. Linst.: From *Gavialis gangeticus.*

(b) Anisakoidea

The members of this family are intestinal parasites frequently transmitted by earthworms (*Porrocaecum*).

Dujardinascaris: At least eleven species from crocodiles (*D. helicina* Baylis, *D. longispicula* Baylis and others) (Fig. 319e).

Multicaecum: Five species from crocodiles.

Polycaecum: *P. gangeticum* Maplestone, a parasite of crocodiles.

Porrocaecum: One species, *P. sulcatum* Baylis in marine turtles.

Terranova crocodili Mosgowy: A parasite of crocodiles.

Angusticaecum: Parasites of crocodiles (*A. holopterum* Baylis) (Fig. 319f) has also been seen in various species of *Testudo* (Baylis, loc. cit.).

Metangusticaecum brasiliense Mosgowy: A parasite of crocodiles.

Amplicaecum: Six species at least have been described from snakes, chameleons, lizards. (*A. africanum* Taylor, *A. alatum* Baylis and others.)

Typhloporus lamellaris Linstow: A parasite of crocodiles.

(c) Trichostrongyloidea

These nematodes, usually large types occurring in mammals, can also infest reptiles. Their life cycles are as yet largely unknown but it can be assumed that, as a rule, the early development takes place in the soil and that the infective stage is that of the third larva.

Oswaldocruzia: Six species in lizards (*O. agamae* Sandground) and snakes (*O. denudata* Rud.)

Herpetostrongylus pythonis Baylis: An intestinal parasite of the python, *H. varani* Baylis.

(d) Trichocephaloidea

Some members of this Superfamily occur in reptiles. The exact mode of development is only known for *Theileriana variabilis* Chapin.

Sclerotrichum echinatum Rud.: A parasite of lizards.

Capillaria: A number of species living in lizards and snakes.

Eucoleus freitaslenti Skrjabin and Schichobalowa: From snakes.

Thominx serpentina Skrjabin and ·Schichobalowa: From *Chelydra serpentina*.

Theileriana variabilis Chapin: From *Testudo denticulata* L.

Sauricola: Two species in chelonians (Fig. 320).

(e) Oxyuroidea

This extremely numerous Superfamily provides about 150 reptilian parasites derived from various genera.

Oxyuris: None definitely described from reptiles. Forstner (1960), however, pictures *O. lata* as a chelonian parasite (Fig. 325, right).

Thelandros: After Skrjabin at least 12 reptilian species, small to medium in size, mostly slender (Fig. 323b).

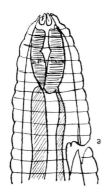 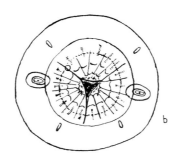 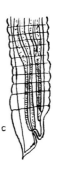

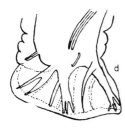

FIG. 320. Trichocephaloidea. *Sauricola sauricola* Chapin. a, anterior extremity. × 60; b, cross section through rostral region. × 240; c , ♀ posterior extremity. × 32; d, Bursa. × 60. (After Chapin from Yorke and Maplestone.)

Parapharyngodon: At least seventeen species living in the gut of lizards, snakes and chelonians (Fig. 321). As typical of the genus may be quoted *P. maplestoni* Chatterji from *Hemidactylus flaviviridis* Rüpp.

Thelastomoides: Three species from tortoises.

Ozolaimus: Two species from *Iguana tuberculata* Laur., *O. megatyphlon* Duj. (Fig. 322a), *O. cirratus* Linstow (Fig. 322b).

Macracis: Two species from lizards, *M. papillosa* Forstner from *Testudo graeca* L.

Travassozolaimus travassosi Vigueras: In chameleons.

Pharyngodon: Large genus. More than thirteen well-defined species occur in saurians. *P. spinicauda* in lizards. (Fig. 323a), *P. mammillatus* Linstow in *Eumeces* spp. (Fig. 321d).

Parathelandros: At least seven species from saurians, particularly geckos.

Spauligodon: At least ten species in saurians, particularly in geckos (Fig. 323c), distinguished by wing-like dilations of the posterior segments.

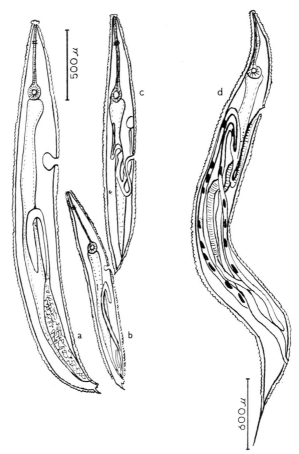

Fig. 321. Oxyuroidea in reptiles. I. a–c, *Parapharyngodon bulbosus* Freitas; a and b, ♂; c, ♀; d, *Pharyngodon mamillatus* Linstow ♀. (From Dollfus, after Skrjabin.)

Tachygonetria: At least twenty well-defined species from saurians and tortoises. *T. vivipara* Wedl (Fig. 323f), *T. dentata* Seurat (Fig. 325, middle), *T. longicollis* Seurat (Fig. 324 left), *T. robusta* Drasche (Fig. 325 left), *T. thapari* Dubiniana (Fig. 327). Most of

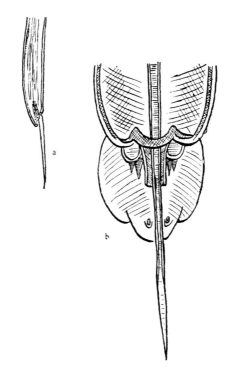

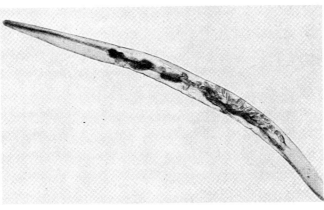

(c)

Fig. 322. Oxyuroidea in reptiles. II. a, *Ozolaimus megatyphlon* Rud.; b, *Ozolaimus cirratus* Linstow. (From Schneider and Linstow in Yorke and Maplestone.) c, *Macracis papillosa* Forstner ♀. × 15. (From Forstner.)

them slender, lancet-shaped medium-sized types without particular distinguishing marks.

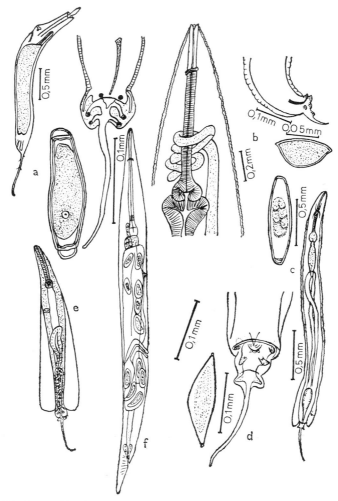

FIG. 323. Oxyuroidea in reptiles. III. a, *Pharyngodon spinicauda* Dies. ♀, egg and posterior extremity of ♂. (After Seurat.) b, *Thelandros hemidactylus* Pathwardhan, anterior extremity, ♂ posterior extremity and egg; c, *Parathelandros mabuyae* Sandground. Egg and ♂; d, *Spauligodon cubensis*. Read and Amrein. Egg and ♂ posterior extremity; e, *Spauligodon mearnsi* Edgerly ♂; f, *Tachygonetria vivipa* a Wedl. ♀. (After Seurat.)

Alaeuris: A few species from tortoises and iguanids (Fig. 326). The males are equipped with very long spiculae.

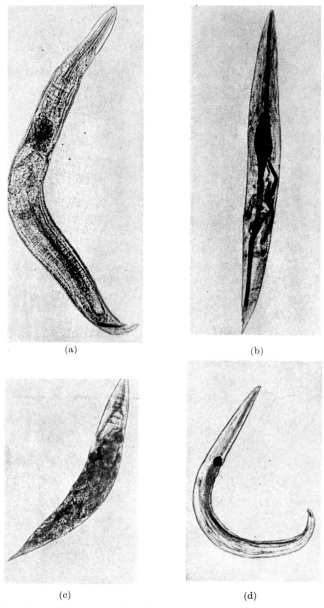

FIG. 324. Oxyuroidea in reptiles. IV. a, c, *Tachygonetria longicollis.* ♀ above, ♀ below. ×21. (After Forstner.) b, d, *Tachygonetria* sp. (= *testudinis* Forstner). ♀ above, ♂ below. (After Forstner.)

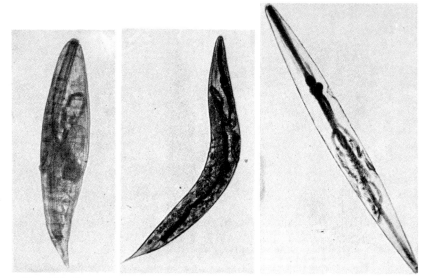

FIG. 325. Oxyuroidea in reptiles. V. Left, *Tachygonetria robusta* Drasche ♀.×21. Middle, *Tachygonetria dentata* Seurat ♀.×21. (After Forstner.) Right, *Oxyuris* (?) *lata* Forstner ♀.×15. (After Forstner.)

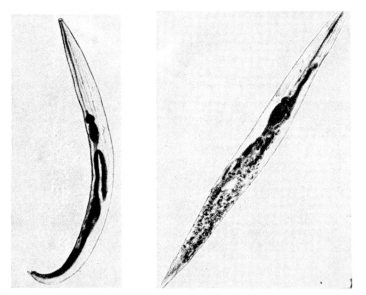

FIG. 326. Oxyuroidea in reptiles. VI. *Alaeuris forcipiformis* Forstner. Left, ♂.×21. Right, ♀.×14. (From Forstner.)

Mehdiella: Parasites of tortoises (Fig. 328).

Paralaeuris dorochila Cuckler from the gut of *Conolophus subcristatus* Gray (Galapagos islands).

Pseudalaeuris: At least sixteen species from saurians and tortoises. *P. expansa* Walton from *Testudo horsfieldi* Gray. The males are recognized by the presence of numerous papilli at the anal extremity (Fig. 327).

Thaparia: A few species from tortoises.

Veversia: A few species from saurians.

Atractis: Parasites of tortoises (Fig. 329).

Labidurus: Parasites of tortoises (Fig. 330a).

Kathlania: Only one species, *K. leptura* Rud. from *Chelonia mydas* L.

Tonaudia: Only one species, *T. tonaudia* Lane, from *Chelonia mydas* L.

Spironoura: Several species from chelonians and snakes.

Zanclophorus: Parasites of chelonians (Fig. 330). *Z. ararath* Massimow.

Cissophyllus: Parasites of chelonians.

(f) Strongyloidea

As a rule parasites of the intestinal tract. Slender types of medium and large size, represented particularly by the Family Diaphanocephalidae genus *Kalicephalus*.

Strongyloides pererai Trav. in *Ophioides striatus* Wagler.

Diaphanocephalus: *D. galeatus* Railliet and Henry from *Tupinambis teguixin* L., *D. diesingi* Freitas and Lent from *Tupinambis nigropunctatus* sp.

Kalicephalus: Numerous genus with over fifty well-determined species from snakes. Typical is the broad shapeless cephalic extremity and the bursa (Fig. 331). Best known: *K. mucronatus* Molin, *K. boae*, Harwood, *K. minutus* Ortlepp, and *K. parvus* Ortlepp.

Occipitodontus: A few species from snakes.

Hexadontophorus: *H. ophisauri* Kreis, from *Ophisaurus* spp.

(g) Cosmocercoidea

Mainly parasites of fish and amphibians. Only a few species in reptilians.

Aplectana amhersti Azim in *Chrysolophus amhersti*.

Aplectana chamaeleonis Travassos in *Chamaeleo fischeri*.

Aplectana hylambatis Trav. in *Leptopelis aubryi* Dum.

Bellaplectana, Neoxysomatium and *Raillietnema* are occasionally found in amphibians and reptiles. *Raillietnema loveridgei* Trav. occurs in *Bdellophis vittatus* Boul., *Neopharyngodon gekko* Chakranarty and Bhaduri in *Gekko gekko* L.

(h) Heterakoidea

Meteterakis: A parasite of amphibians mainly. In reptilians we find:

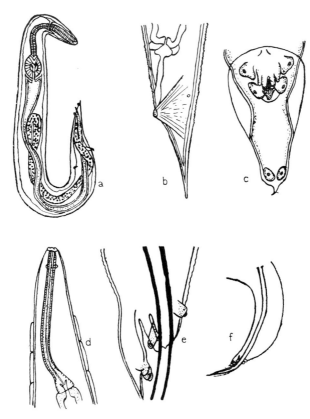

FIG. 327. Oxyuroidea in reptiles. VII. a–c, *Pseudalaeuris expansa* Rees. ♀ and ♂ posterior extremities. (From Rees.) d–f, *Alaeuris conspicua* Ortlepp. Anterior and posterior extremity of ♂ seen from above and sideways. (After Ortlepp.)

M. cophotis Freitas: In Agamids.

M. longispiculata Inglis (= *Spinicauda longicauda longispiculata* Baylis): In *Gekko gekko* L. (Fig. 332h–i).

M. louisi Inglis: In saurians.

M. mabuyae Inglis: In *Mabuya carinata* Schn.

M. varani Skrjabin, Schichobalowa and Lagodowskaja (= *Africana varani* Maplestone): In *Varanus bengalensis*.

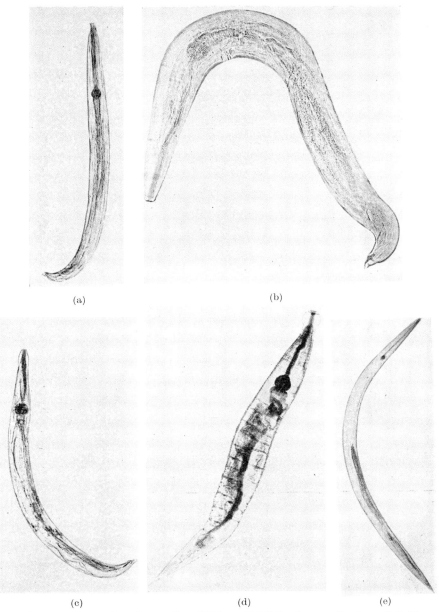

(a)   (b)

(c)   (d)   (e)

FIG. 328. Oxyuroidea in reptiles. VIII. a, *Mehdiella hamosa* Forstner ♂. × 30; b, *Mehdiella cordata* Forstner ♂. × 72. (After Forstner.) c, *Mehdiella uncinata* Drasche ♂; d, *Mehdiella uncinata* ♀. Both × 25; e, *Mehdiella microstoma* Seurat ♂. × 15. (After Forstner.)

Spinicauda

At least seven species in saurians and chameleons. *Sp. spinicauda* Olfers occurs in *Podicnema teguexin* L. (Fig. 332a-d), *Sp. sonsinoi* Linstow in lizards and in *Chamaeleo vulgaris* L.

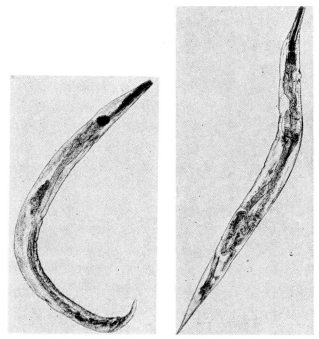

FIG. 329. Oxyuroidea in reptiles. IX. *Atractis dactylura* Duj. Left, ♂; right, ♀. × 30. (After Forstner.)

Africana

Three species in tortoises (*A. africana* Trav. Fig. 332k-l) and chameleons. (*A. acuticeps* Trav.)

Strongyluris

At least twenty-three species in saurians, chameleons and snakes.

St. brevicaudata Müller: Occurs in *Agama agama agama* L. and in *Chamaeleo dilepis* Leach (Fig. 332e-g).

St. chamaeleonis Baylis and Daubney: In *Chamaeleo vulgaris* L.

St. ornata Railliet and Henry: In *Stellio vulgaris* Latr.

Moaciria alvarengai Freitas: Occurs in *Lygosoma maculata* Blyth.

Ganguleterakis: According to Kreis (1940) some representatives of the genus parasitize reptilians.

(i) Camallanoidea

Parasites of stomach and intestine, mostly medium sized worms. *Camallanus*. Several species in chelonians.

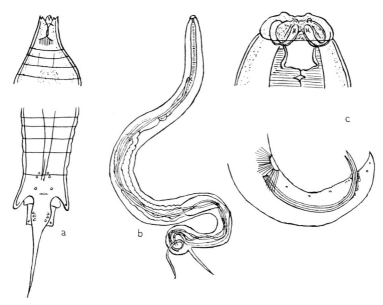

FIG. 330. Oxyuroidea in reptiles. X. a, *Labiduris gulosa* Rud. Anterior extremity. × 80. Posterior extremity of ♂. × 66. (After Schneider from Yorke and Maplestone.) b, *Tonaudia tonaudia* Lane ♂. × 10. (After Lane from Yorke and Maplestone.) c, *Zanclophorus annandalei* Baylis and Daubney. Anterior extremity above; ♂ posterior extremity below. × 18. (From Yorke and Maplestone.)

(j) Spiruroidea

A varied group of nematodes which change hosts during development. While fish, aquatic reptiles and amphibians ingest the larval stages of these worms when feeding on copepodes, terrestrial reptiles infect themselves through feeding on beetles and other insects. The reptiles function mainly as intermediate hosts, the final hosts being dogs.

Spiroxys: Several species in the stomach of chelonians.

Spirocerca: *S. lupi* Rud. The African lizard *Eremias arguta* ingests the larva by feeding on a beetle which serves as temporary transport host. The larva undergoes a resting period in the peritoneal cavity of the reptile. The final stage develops in a dog.

Physaloptera: Numerous species in the stomach and the gut of saurians, chameleons and snakes.

Abbreviata: Parasites of stomach and gut of saurians.

Skrjabinoptera: Particularly *S. colubri*, a common parasite of snakes. Other species in lizards.

Thubunaea: *T. pudica* Seurat, a parasite of chameleons (Fig. 333d-e).

Proleptus: A parasite of chelonians.

Gnathostoma: Parasites of crocodiles. First intermediate host: copepodes. Second: fish or amphibians, also reptiles.

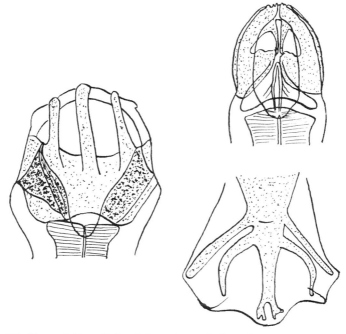

Fig. 331. Strongyloidea. *Kalicephalus minutus* Ortlepp. Left, Anterior extremity. × 240. Right above, Anterior extremity sideways. × 200. Below, Bursa. × 200. (After Baylis and Daubney from Yorke and Maplestone.)

Larval stages of *Gnathostoma* species are frequently seen in reptiles (Fig. 333f). For details see Daengsvang (1949) and Miyazaki and Ash (1959). Ash (1962) quotes the following reptiles as being natural second intermediate hosts of *Gnathostoma procyonis* Chandler: the snakes *Agkistrodon piscivorus* Lac., *Natrix r. rhombifera* Hallowell, *Natrix sipedon* L., *Lampropeltis getulus* L.; the chelonians *Kinosternon subrubrum hippocrepis* Gray, *Terrapene carolina major* Agassiz and *Alligator mississippiensis* Daud. The larvae, about 1 mm long, are found free in the tissue of the reptiles. The first intermediate hosts are

Cyclops species. The mature worms are found within small tumours of the gastric wall of herons.

Dermal oedema of the face and the limbs in Siam have been found to be caused by *Gnathostoma spinigerum* Owen (Daengsvang, 1949). Again *Cyclops* species function as first intermediate hosts. The second

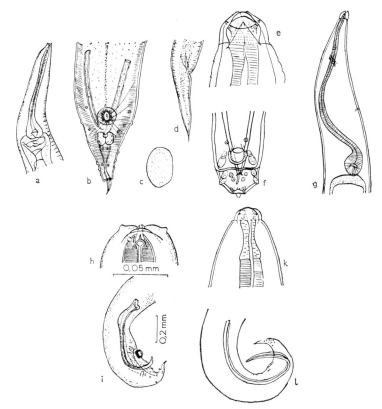

Fig. 332. Heterakoidea. a–d, *Spinicauda spinicauda* Olfers. a, Anterior extremity; b, ♂ posterior extremity; c, egg; d, ♀ posterior extremity. (After Travassos from Yorke and Maplestone.) e–g, *Strongyluris brevicaudata* Müller; e, anterior extremity. × 165; f, ♂ posterior extremity. × 45; g, anterior extremity. × 23. (From Yorke and Maplestone.) h–i, *Meteterakis longispiculata* Inglis; h, anterior extremity; i, ♂ posterior extremity; k–l, *Africana africana* Travassos; k, anterior extremity; l, ♂ posterior extremity. × 38. (From Yorke and Maplestone.)

hosts are fish and aquatic snakes of undetermined species, which carry the parasite in the muscular and intestinal tissues. People are warned therefore not to eat freshwater creatures raw or insufficiently cooked.

Tanqua: Parasites of varanids and snakes. Development as in the previous genus. *T. anomala* Linstow (Fig. 333b-c).

Hedruris: Gastric parasites of chelonians.

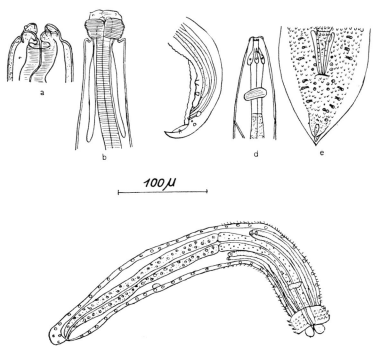

100 µ

FIG. 333. Spiruroidea. a, *Spiroxys contorta*, anterior extremity. × 80. (After Baylis and Lane from Yorke and Maplestone.) b–c, *Tanqua anomala* Linstow, anterior extremity, ♂ posterior extremity. Both × 28. (After Yorke and Maplestone.) d–e, *Thubunaea pudica* Seurat, anterior extremity and ♂ posterior extremity. Both × 85. (After Seurat from Yorke and Maplestone.) f, Third larval stage of *Gnathostoma procyonis* Chandler from a Cyclops sp. (After Ash.)

Pulmonary Nematodes

Reptilian lungs may be infested by representatives of the Order Rhabdiasiodea or by *Pneumonema tiliquae* Johnston, a member of the Family Rictulariidae.

It is a peculiarity of the Rhabdiasioidea that they alternate between free-living and parasitic forms. The sexually mature free-living form produces filariform juveniles which search for the chance to penetrate the skin of a suitable host. Having gained access by this way or by becoming actually a part of the food on which the host feeds, the filariform worms find their way to the lungs. In the lungs the worms develop into hermaphrodites. Fertilized eggs are swallowed and hatch in the colon, producing rhabdiform larvae which are voided with the faeces and so deposited on the soil where they grow to sexual maturity.

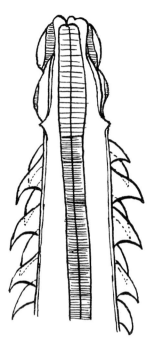

FIG. 334. *Pneumonia tiliquae* Johnston. Anterior extremity. × 215. (From Yorke and Maplestone.)

Rhabdiasioidea: Worms of the genus *Rhabdias* may be found in the lungs of chameleons, slow-worms and snakes. Sprehn (1961) mentions the species *Rhabdias dujardini* Maupas-Seurat and *Rh. entomelas* Duj. from *Anguis fragilis* L. and *Rh. fuscovenosa* Railliet from *Natrix natrix* L.

Pneumonema tiliquae Johnston (Fig. 334) is a pulmonary parasite of *Tiliqua scincoides* White.

Nematodes of the Circulatory and Lymphatic System

Nematodes parasitizing the circulatory and lymphatic systems of reptilians belong to the Superfamilies Dracunculoidea and Filarioidea. They affect particularly the subcutaneous connective tissue where they cause tumours, oedema and inflammation.

Dracunculoidea

Dracunculus: Five species, some of appreciable size. The juvenile larvae live free at the bottom of ponds where they are taken up by copepodes which are, in turn, eaten by the final host.

Dracunculus medinensis L.: The guinea worm, well-known in human pathology, may occasionally also be found in the dermis of reptilians. Desportes (1938) found the closely allied species *Filaria oesophagea* Polonio (1895) in *Natrix natrix persa* Pallas. He found in the mediastinum juvenile females of 27–85 mm length, adult females of 28–44 mm length, males of 11–20 mm and embryos of

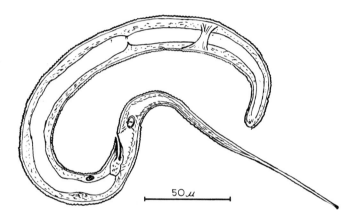

FIG. 335. Embryo of *Dracunculus oesophageus* Polonio. (After Desportes.)

just under 0·5 mm (Fig. 335). Experiments determined *Macrocyclops fuscus* Jur. as intermediate host. Desportes named the species *Dracunculus oesophageus* Polonio.

D. globocephalus Mackie: Occurs in *Chelydra serpentina* L.

D. houdemeri Hsü: In *Natrix piscator* Schn.

D. dahomensis Neumann: In *Python* spp. *D. ophidensis* Brackett in *Thamnophis sirtalis* L.

Even the expert may have difficulties in distinguishing between the various *Dracunculus* species quoted. Mirza (1958) suggests assigning to one and the same species all Dracunculids found in snakes.

Filarioidea

Short, slender worms transmitted by arthropods, mosquitoes and mites. Reptilia may harbour sexually mature forms as well as juvenile

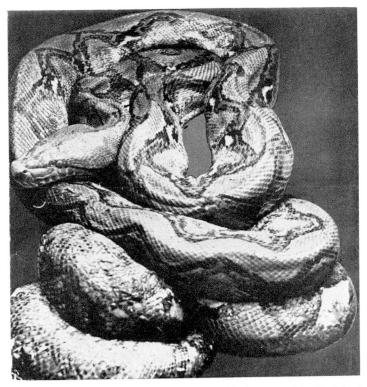

FIG. 336. *Python reticulatus* Schneider with dermal lesions caused by filarial infection. (Photo.: W. Frank.)

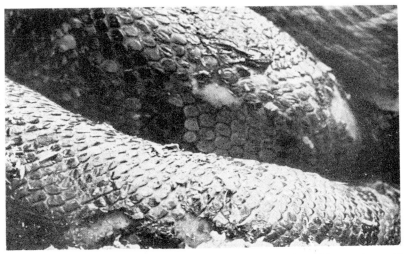

FIG. 337. Part of Fig. 336 at higher magnification, showing dermal destruction and loss of scales. (Photo.: W. Frank.)

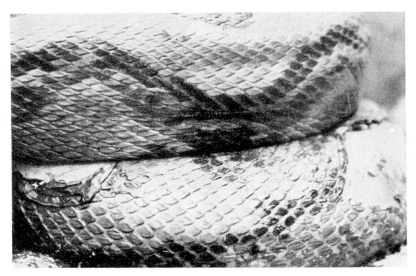

Fig. 338. *Python reticulatus* Schneider. Early dermal destruction caused by filarial infection. On the right is an old wound. (Photo.: W. Frank.)

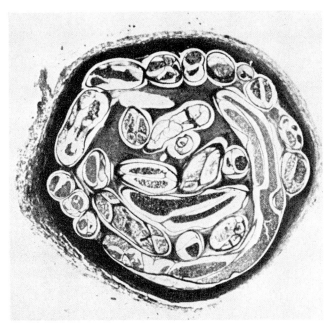

Fig. 339. Section through the mesenteric artery of *Python molurus bivittatus* Kühl filled with adult filarial worms of *Macdonaldius oschei* Chabaud and Frank. (Photo.: W. Frank)

larvae, microfilariae which, occurring in large numbers may block both circulatory and lymphatic vessels causing thrombosis and oedema.

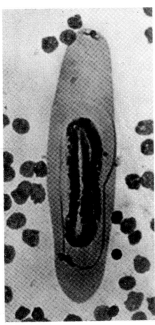

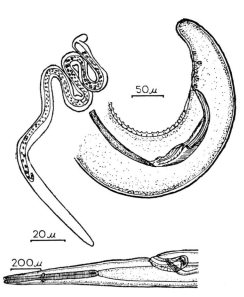

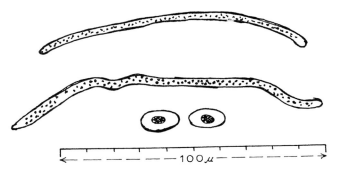

FIG. 340. *Macdonaldius oschei* Chabaud and Frank. Microfilaria in the vein of *Epicrates cenchris* L. Stained Giemsa. (Photo.: W. Frank.)

FIG. 341. *Macdonaldius andersoni* Chabaud and Frank. Above left, Microfilaria; right, posterior extremity. Below, anterior extremity. From Chabaud and Frank.

FIG. 342. Microfilariae of *Thamugadia physignathi* Cleland from the brain of *Physignathus lesueuri* Gray. Drawn by microprojection. (E. Elkan.)

Frank (1962) reports on the death of pythons in the Stuttgart Zoo. The animals died with large dermal lesions (Figs. 336–338) and the post-mortem examination revealed the presence of several hundreds of mature filaria in the mesenteric arteries as well as numerous "sheathed" stages of the microfilarial type *Macdonaldius oschei* Chabaud and Frank (Figs. 339–341). Altogether at least twelve genera are, with numerous species, represented in reptilians. Only in three of them has it been possible to determine the whole life cycle. The adult worms are mostly of medium length. In *Macdonaldius oschei* the females measure 62 mm; in *M. andersoni* 50 mm; the males 33 and 22 mm respectively. The caudal extremity of the males is armed with a number of spiculae and papillae. The diameter of the microfilaria in both species is 0·2 mm.

One of us (E. E.) had the opportunity of studying a case of extensive microfilarial infection in an Australian water dragon (*Physignathus lesueuri*) which died after 9 years of captivity in an English animal collection. The large, pale, friable and oedematous fat body contained numerous microfilaria (Fig. 342). These were, in fact, present in the blood vessels, particularly in the capillaries of every organ, and were particularly numerous in the brain, where some of them could be seen to lie outside the capillaries embedded in the brain substance itself. In spite of this massive infestation no organ showed any cellular reaction or signs of necrobiosis. The water dragon must have been infected before it reached England and must therefore have lived with the infection for at least 9 years, which makes it doubtful whether the filariae were the sole cause of death. They had, on the other hand, caused extensive degenerative changes in the kidneys (Fig. 343) where the parenchymatous epithelium had almost completely disappeared leaving only the meshwork of the interstitial reticulum behind. The number of worms in the renal capillaries, however, was rather smaller than that in the brain where no evidence of local damage could be demonstrated (Fig. 345). The parasite was determined as *Thamugadia physignathi* Cleland, described from the liver and the mesenteric vessels of *Physignathus lesueuri* Gray by Johnston (1912), Johnston and Cleland (1911) and by Johnston and Mawson (1953). The transmitting vector, probably a mosquito, is not known yet.

Hastospiculum: At least four species in the blood vessels of varanids and snakes.

Foleyella: Some species parasitize the blood of lizards. A well-known species is, for instance, *F. candazei* Fraipont from *Uromastix acanthinurus* Bell and *F. agamae* Rodhain from Agamids. W. Frank, in a personal communication to R.-Klinke (1962), reported

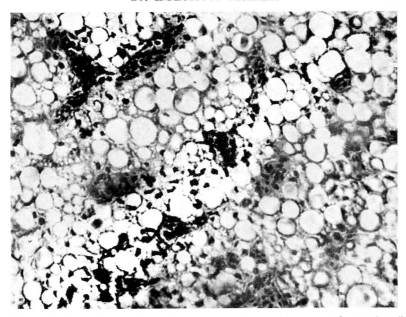

FIG. 343. Kidney of a specimen of *Physignathus lesueuri*, the water dragon, heavily infected with microfilaria of *Thamugadia physignathi*. Renal parenchyma almost completely destroyed.

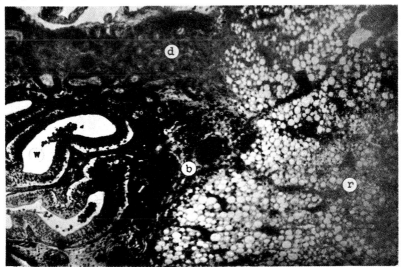

FIG. 344. As Fig. 343, showing the borderline between normal (left), and degenerate (right) tissue. *b*, Blood vessels; *d*, renal tubules; *r*, degenerate renal tissue; *w*, Wolffian duct. (Photo.: E. Elkan.)

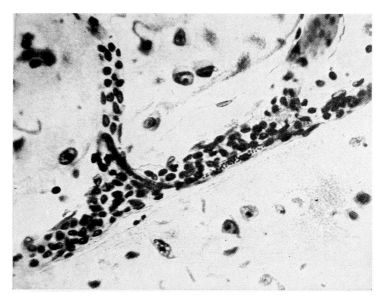

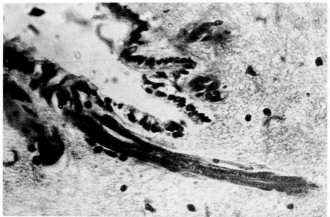

FIG. 345. Microfilaria of *Thamugadia physignathi* Cleland in the brain of *Physignathus lesueuri*. Intravascular worms (above), extravascular worms (below).

having again found *Foleyella furcata* Linstow 1899 in *Chamaeleo oustaleti* Mcqu.

Oswaldofilaria: Parasites of saurians and crocodiles. Mackerras (1953) determined the mosquitoes *Culex annulirostris* Skuse and *Culex fatigans* Wied as vectors of *Oswaldofilaria chlamydosauri* Breinl.

Macdonaldius: Five species in snakes, iguanids and *Heloderma*. Frank (1962) determined the mite *Ornithodoros talaje* Guérin and Méneville as vector of *Madonaldius oschei* Chabaud and Frank. For a detailed description see the original publication (Figs. 339–341).

Saurofilaria: Parasites of Mexican saurians.

Thamugadia: Parasites of saurians. cf. the earlier description of an infection of *Physignathus lesueuri* Gray.

Pseudothamugadia: Parasites of reptiles.

Saurositus: Haemoparasites of agamids (Macfie, 1924).

Conispiculum: Parasites of saurians. Pandit, Pandit and Iyer (1929) determined *Culex fatigans* as vector of *Conispiculum flavescens* P. P. and I.

Piratuba and *Cardianema*: Rarer haemoparasites of reptilians.

Micropleura: Haemofilaria of crocodiles. *M. vazi* Trav. in the peritoneal cavity of *Caiman sclerops* Gray.

The number of helminthic species found in reptiles closely approaches that of fish. The number of genera is slightly larger. Yamaguti (1961) lists:

28 Families of digenetic trematodes;
6 Families of cestodes;
31 Families of nematodes.

The nematodes embraced 105 genera with 583 species.

REFERENCES

Ash, L. R. and Beaver, P. C. (1962). A restudy of *Ophidascaris labiatopapillosa* occurring in the stomach of N. American snakes. *J. Parasit.* **48**, (Suppl.), 41.

Ash, L. R. (1962). Development of *Gnathostoma procyonis* Chandler 1942, in the first and second intermediate hosts. *J. Parasit.* **48**, 298–305.

Baylis, H. A. (1921). On the classification of the ascaridae. II. The *Polydelphis* group with some account of other ascarids parasitic in snakes. *Parasitology* **12**, 411–426.

Baylis, H. A. (1929). Some new parasitic nematodes and cestodes from Java. *Parasitology* **21**, 256–265.

Baylis, H. A. and Daubney, R. (1922). Reports on the parasitic nematodes in the collection of the Zoological Survey of India. *Mem. Ind. Mus.* **7**, 263–347.

Caballero, E. C. (1954). Nematodes de los Reptiles de Mexico. XI. Nuevo genero y nueva especie de Filaria de Iguanidos. *Rev. Parasit.* **15**, 305–313.

Chabaud, A. G. and Frank, W. (1961). Nouvelle filaire parasite des artères de pythons: *Macdonaldius oschei* n. sp. (Nematodes, Onchocercidae). *Z. Parasitenk.* **20**, 434–439.

Chabaud, A. G. and Frank, W. (1961). Nouvelle filaire, parasite des artères de l'*Heloderma suspectum* Cope: *Macdonaldius andersoni* n. sp. (Nematodes, Onchocercidae). *Ann. Parasit. hum. comp.* **36**, 127–136.

Chabaud, A. G. and Frank, W. (1961). Les filaires de l'Héloderme. Note additive. *Ann. Parasit. hum. comp.* **36**, 804–805.

Chitwood, B. G. and Chitwood, M. B. (1950). "An Introduction to Nematology." Washington.

Daengsvang, S. (1949). Human gnathostomiasis in Siam, with reference to the method of prevention. *J. Parasit.* **35**, 116–121.

Desportes, C. (1938). *Filaria oesophagea* Polonio 1895, parasite de la couleuvre d'Italie, est un Dracunculus très voisin de la filaire de medine. *Ann. Parasit. hum. comp.* **16**, 305–326.

Edgerley, R. H. (1952). Two new species of Nematoda, *Strongyluris riversidensis* and *Pharyngodon mearnsi* from Lizard *Streptosaurus mearnsi*. *Trans. Amer. micr. Soc.* **71**, 288–292.

Fitzsimmons, W. M. (1958). *Saurositus macfiei* sp. nov., a filarioid parasite of the lizard *Agama mossambica mossambica* Peters. *Ann.trop. Med. Par.* **52**, 257–260.

Forstner, M. J. (1960). Ein Beitrag zur Kenntnis parasitischer Nematoden aus griechischen Landschildkröten. *Z. Parasitenk.* **20**, 1–22.

Hsü, H. F. (1933). On *Dracunculus houdemeri* n. sp., *Dracunculus globocephalus* and *Dracunculus medinensis*. *Z. Parasitenk.* **6**, 101–118.

Inglis, W. G. (1958). A revision of the nematode genus *Meteterakis* Karve, 1930. *Parasitology* **48**, 9–31.

Johnston, T. H. and Cleland, B. (1911). The haematozoa of Australian reptilia. *Proc. Linn. Soc. N.S. Wales* **36**, 479–491.

Johnston, T. H. (1912). Notes on some Entozoa. *Proc. Roy. Soc. Queensland* **24**, 63–91.

Johnston, T. H. (1912). A census of Australian reptilian Entozoa. *Proc. Roy. Soc. Queensland* **24**, 233–249.

Johnston, T. H. and Mawson, P. M. (1943). Remarks on some nematodes from Australian reptiles. *Trans. Roy. Soc. S. Austr.* **67**, 183–186.

Kreis, H. A. (1940). Ein neuer parasitischer Nematode aus *Corucia zebrata* (Scincidae, Reptilia). *Ganguleterakis triaculeatus* n. sp. *Z. Parasitenk.* **6**, 332–338.

Kreis, H. A. (1940). Beiträge zur Kenntnis parasitischer Nematoden. IX. Parasitische Nematoden aus dem Naturhistorischen Museum Basel. *Zbl. Bakt. Orig.* **145**, 163–208.

Macfie, J. W. S. (1924). *Saurositus agamae* n. g., n. sp., a filarioid parasite of the lizard *Agama colonorum*. *Ann. trop. Med. Par.* **18**, 409–412.

Mackerras, M. F. (1953). Lizard Filaria: Transmission by mosquitoes of *Oswaldofilaria chlamydosauri* Breinl. (Nematoda, Filarioidea). *Parasitology* **43**, 1–3.

Mirza, M. B. (1958). On *Dracunculus* Reichard, 1759 and its species. *Z. Parasitenk.* **18**, 44–47.

Miyazaki, J. and Ash, L. R. (1959). On the gnathostome larvae found from snakes in New Orleans, U.S.A. (In Japanese.) *Jap. J. Parasit.* **8**, 351–352.

Ortlepp, R. J. (1933a). *Ozolaimus megatyphlon* Rud., a little known helminth from *Iguana tuberculata*. *Onderst. J. Vet. Sci. An. Ind.* **1**, 99–114.

Ortlepp, R. J. (1937b). On some South African reptilian oxyurids. *J. Vet. Sci. An. Ind.* **1**, 99–114.

Pandit, C. G., Pandit, S. R. and Iyer, P. V. S. (1929). The development of the filaria *Conispiculum guindiensis* (1929) in *Culex fatigans*, with a note on the transmission of the infection. *Ind. J. med. Res.* **17**, 421–429.

Patwardhan, S. S. (1935). Nematodes from the common wall lizard *Hemidactylus flaviviridis* Rüppel. *Proc. Ind. Acad. Sci.* **1**, (7) 376–380.

Read, C. P. and Amrein, Y. U. (1935). North American nematodes of the genus *Pharyngodon* Diesing. (Oxyuridae). *J. Parasit.* **39**, 365–370.

Rees, F. G. (1935). Two new species of *Tachygonetria* from the Indian tortoise *Testudo horsfieldi* Gray. *Proc. zool. Soc. Lond.* **3**, 599–603.

Sandground, J. H. (1936). Scientific results of an expedition to Rain Forest Regions in Eastern Africa. VI. Nematoda. *Bull. Mus. comp. Zool.* **79**, 341–366.

Seurat, L. G. (1912). Sur les Oxyures de *Uromastix acanthinurus* Bell. *C.R. Soc. Biol., Paris* **73**, 223–226.

Seurat, L. G. (1914). Sur un cas d'Endotokie Matricide chez un Oxyure. *C.R. Soc. Biol., Paris* **76**, 850–852.

Shad, A. G. (1963). Niche diversification in a parasitic species flock. *Nature, Lond.* **198**, 404–406.

Skrjabin, K. J. (1960). "Ossnowy Nematodologii." Moscow (in Russian).

Smith, A. J. (1910). A new filarial species (*F. mitchelli* n. sp.) found in *Heloderma suspectum*, and its larvae in a tick parasite upon the Gila Monster, with remarks upon ticks as possible intermediate hosts in filariasis. *Univ. Pennsylvan. Med. Bull.* **23**, 487–497.

Sonsino, P. (1889). Studi e notizie elminthologiche. *Atti Soc. tosc. sci. nat.* **6**, 224–237.

Waitz, J. A. (1961). Parasites of Idaho Reptiles. *J. Parasit.* **47**, 51.

Yamaguti, S. (1961). "Systema Helminthum", Vol. III. Interscience, London-New York.

Yorke, W. and Maplestone, P. A. (1926). "The Nematode Parasites of Vertebrates." Churchill, London.

H. Leeches

Leeches are mainly found on turtles and crocodiles. A review of the species likely to be encountered has been given by Autrum (1936). The genus *Haementeria* is particularly well represented with fifteen species from turtles and two from crocodiles. In Europe we find *Haementeria costata* Fr. Müller on *Emys orbicularis* L., in E. Asia and N. America *H. rugosa* Vervil. On crocodiles we find *H. fimbriata* Johansson (*Crocodilus niloticus* L.) and *H. maculata* Weber on Brazilian crocodiles. All these species seem to be exclusively adapted to life on one specific host; the finding of *Haementeria okadai* Oka, which ordinarily parasitizes frogs, in the mouth of a turtle, may have been a chance event. An interesting species is *Haementeria costata* Müller (= *Placobdella stepanowi* Blanchard) which transmits the blood parasite *Haemogregarina stepanowi* Danilewsky.

The species *Hemiclepsis marginata* O. F. Müller, on the other hand, which occurs from Europe to Japan, has a wide spectrum of hosts including besides fish and larval amphibians the turtle *Chinemys reevesii* Gray.

Actinobdella annectens Moore has been found on the common snapping turtle (*Chelydra serpentina* L.).

Members of the genus *Ozobranchus* not only suck blood like *Haementeria* but also transmit various diseases. *Ozobranchus shipleyi* Harding for instance has been found to transmit *Haemogregarina nicoriae* Castellani and Wiley in *Geoemyda trijuga* Schweigger. Other species of *Ozobranchus* are found on marine turtles and freshwater turtles as well as on crocodiles.

Nigrelli and Smith (1943) studied the histological evidence of the damage caused by attacks of leeches when they found *Ozobranchus* associated with fibroepitheliomata in the marine turtle *Chelonia mydas* L.

REFERENCES

Autrum, H. (1936). Hirudineen. Pt. I. *In* Bronn's "Klassen und Ordnungen des Tierreichs." Quelle and Meyer, Leipzig.

Nigrelli, R. F. and Smith, G. M. (1943). The occurrence of leeches, *Ozobranchus branchiatus*, on fibroepithelial tumours of marine turtles *Chelonia mydas*. *Zoologica* **28**, 107–108.

I. Mites (Acarina)

Mites are regarded with great apprehension by the herpetologist both as parasites and as transmitters of diseases. Unfortunately they occur in considerable numbers of reptiles. Some of them limit themselves to one or a few hosts, others show no sign of discrimination. One group, whose final hosts are mammals, pass their juvenile stages on reptilians. The mites fasten themselves in those areas of the skin most suitable for their requirements. Sometimes we may find them under scales, in the axilla, in the inguinal region around the root of the tail, sometimes around the eyes. Some species even penetrate the lungs of snakes. Epidemics of mite invasion occur particularly where many Reptilia are kept in close confinement. The situation can become very serious since the life of the host is threatened if the loss of blood caused by the mites is too severe (Fig. 346).

Approximately 250 different species of mites have so far been described, the commonest being *Ophionyssus natricis* Mégnin which attacks snakes.

In dealing with the individual species we follow the survey of Baker and Wharton (1952).

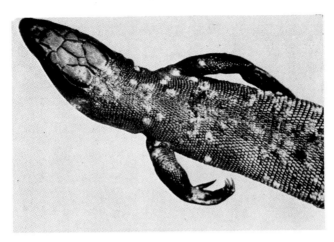

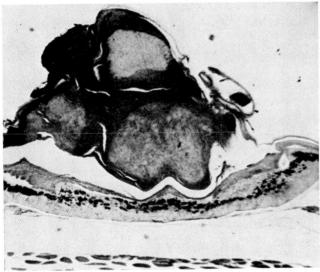

FIG. 346. A specimen of *Lacerta viridis* which was heavily infested with ticks. Above, Anterior part of the lizard showing dermal lesions. Below, Section through the skin showing excessive keratosis. (Photo.: E. Elkan.)

Mesostigmata

Heterozerconidae

Heterozercon oudemansi Finnegan (1931), found as an external parasite on a tropical snake.

Entonyssidae

Parasites of the trachea and the lungs of snakes. Fain (1961) gave a detailed description of these species and revised the family. He found 2% of all snakes investigated infested with these mites. According to

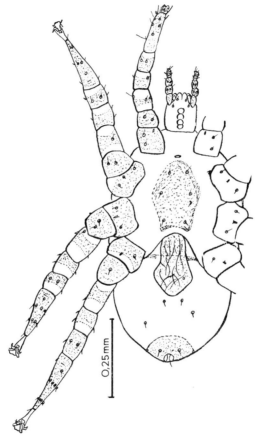

0.25 mm

FIG. 347. *Entonyssus colubri* Hubbard. (After Fain, 1961.)

the state of development, larvae, protonymphs and deutonymphs are distinguished. The mode of transmission has not been determined but nymphs are more numerous in the trachea than in the lungs.

Entonyssus. Six species in Asia and N. America.

E. *halli* Ewing: From *Crotalus* spp. in Texas, particularly *Crotalus cinereus* Le Conte.

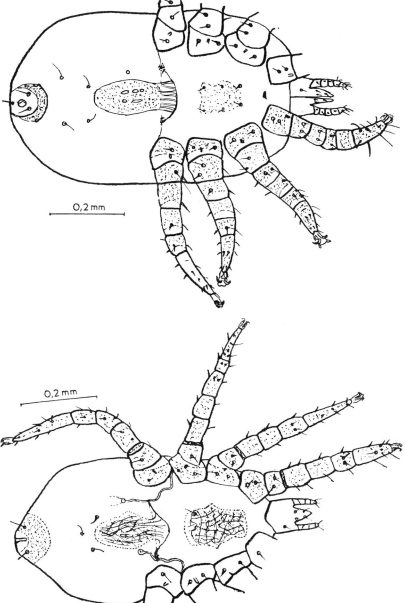

FIG. 348. Left, *Hamertonia radfordi* Fain. Right, *Entophiophaga natriciterei* Fain. (Both from Fain, 1961.)

E. rileyi Ewing: From a *Crotalus* sp. (*Crotalus cinereus* Le Conte) in
Texas.

E. colubri Hubbard comb. Fain: From *Coluber flagellum flaviventris*
Hallowell, *Coluber constrictor constrictor* L., *C. c. foxi* Baird and
Girard (Fig. 347).

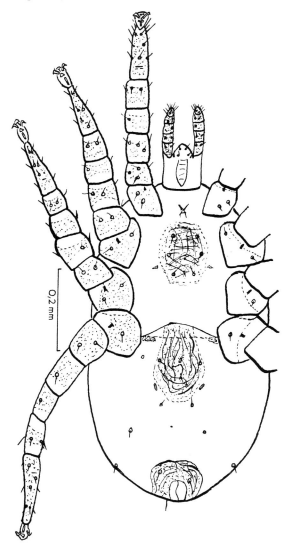

0,2 mm

Fig. 349. *Entophionyssus glasmacheri* Vitzthum. (After Fain, 1961.)

E. asiaticus Fain: From *Natrix chrysarga* Schl., *N. subtruncata* Schl.

E. philippinensis Fain: From *Fordonia leucobalia* Schl. and *Natrix piscator* Schn.

E. javanicus Fain: From *Natrix vittata* L.

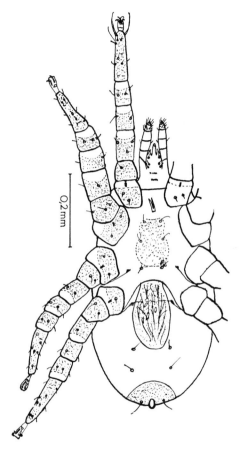

FIG. 350. *Viperacarus europaeus* Fain. (From Fain, 1961.)

Hamertonia bedfordi Radford: From *Dendroaspis angusticeps* Smith.

H. psammophis Till: From *Psammophis s. sibilans* L., *Rhamphiophis oxyrhynchus garambensis* Witte, *Meizodon coronatus* Schl. and *Dromophis lineatus* Dum. and Bibr.

H. radfordi Fain: From *Gastropyxis smaragdina* Schl. (Fig. 348, left).

Entophiophaga congolensis Fain: From *Dasypeltis scaber* L. and *Crotaphopeltis hotamboeia* Laur.

E. scaphiophis Fain: From *Scaphiophis a. albopunctata* Peters.

E. natriciterei Fain: From *Natriciteres o. olivacea* Peters (Fig. 348, right).

E. colubricola Fain: From *Coluber jugularis caspius* Gmelin.

Entophionyssus hamertoni Radford: From *Thamnophis sirtalis parietalis* Say and *T. s. sirtalis* L.

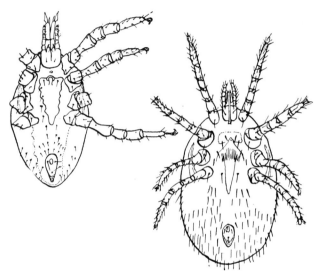

Fig. 351. *Ophionyssus natricis* Mégnin. Left, ♂. (After Radford.) Right, ♀. (After Hirst.)

E. glasmacheri Vitzthum comb. Fain: From *Elaphe quadrivittata* Holbrook, *E. guttata* L., *E. obsoleta* Say and *Pituophis sayi* Schl. (Fig. 349).

E. natricis Keegan comb. Fain: From *Natrix sipedon* L.

E. fragilis Keegan comb. Fain: From *Lampropeltis getulus* L.

E. heterodontos Keegan comb. Fain: From *Heterodon contortrix* L., *Heterodon platyrhinos* Cathesby and *Lampropeltis calligaster* Hln.

Viperacarus europaeus Fain: From *Vipera berus* L. (Fig. 350).

Cobranyssus schoutedeni Radford comb. Fain: From *Naja tripudians fasciatus* Gray.

Pneumophionyssus aristoterisi Fonseca: From *Erythrolamprus aesculapii* L.

Entophioptes liophis Fain: From *Liophis anomalus* Gthr.

Dermanyssidae

The Dermanyssidae are ectoparasites of saurians and snakes. Only *Mabuyonyssus* parasitizes the nostrils.

The commonest blood-sucking tick of snakes, usually found under the scales, is *Ophionyssus* (= *Serpenticola*) *natricis* Mégnin (Gervais) (= *serpentium* Hirst) (Fig. 351).

This tick, which feeds on the blood of snakes, is not only the nightmare of the herpetologist, on occasion it even infests humans. It has been reported (Privorn and Samsinak, 1958) that workers employed in a laboratory where many snakes were kept began to suffer from intense itching followed by the appearance of small boils. Schweizer (1952) tested various substances designed to kill the mites and to disinfect the cages. The most suitable of these proved to be paradichlorbenzol which is used in varying doses according to the species and the size of the snakes. Some snakes react by showing a transient form of paralysis while under treatment. A mixture of castor oil and 90% alcohol in equal parts has also been used successfully.

Ophionyssus variabilis Zemskaya: From *Echis carinata* Schn.

Neoliponyssus gordonensis Hirst: From *Mabuya quinquestriata* Lichtenst.

Neoliponyssus lacertinus Berlese: Occurs on lizards.

N. monodi Hirst: Occurs on *Acanthodactylus* spp.

N. saurarum Oudemans: Occurs on lizards.

Steatonyssus arabicus Hirst: Occurs on *Agama adramitana*.

Mabuyonyssus freedmanni Till was found on the head of *Mabuya quinquetaeniata margaritifer* Peters. Fain (1961) suggests that the usual seat of infection is the nostril.

Omentolaelaptidae

Omentolaelaps mehelyae Fain (Fig. 352) occurs under ventral and ventro-lateral scales of *Mehelya capensis savorgnani* Mocquard and *M. poensis* Smith in the Congo.

Laelaptidae

Ophidilaelaps imphalensis Radford (1947).

Haemolaelaps natricis Feider and Solomon: From *Natrix natrix* L.

Ixodorhynchus liponyssoides Ewing: From *colubrid* snakes.

I. johnstoni Fain: From *Heterodon p. platyrhinos* Latr.

I. leptodeirae Fain: From *Leptodeira maculata* Hallowell.

I. cubanensis Fain: From *Liophis andreae* Reinhardt.

Ixobioides butantanensis Fonseca: From colubrid snakes (Fig. 353).

I. fonsecae Fain: From *Xenodon guentheri* Boul.

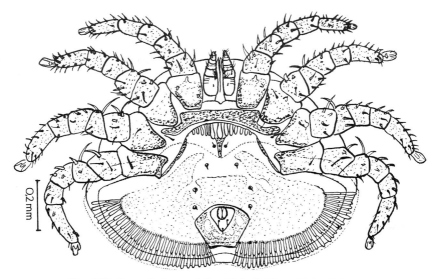

FIG. 352. *Omentolaelaps mehelyae* Fain ♀. (From Fain, 1961.)

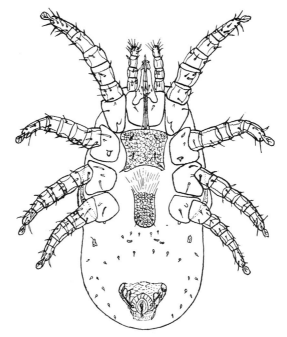

FIG. 353. *Ixodobioides butantanensis* Fonseca ♀. (After Fonseca.)

Hemilaelaps triangulus Ewing: From colubrid snakes, South U.S.A.

H. javanensis Fain: From *Lycodon subcinctus* Boie.

H. farrieri Tibbets: From colubrid snakes, Africa.

H. congolensis Fain: From *Causus rhombeatus* Licht.

H. causicola Fain: From *Causus rhombeatus* Lichtst.

H. dipsadoboae Fain: From *Dipsadoboa unicolor* Guenther.

H. radfordi Feider and Solomon: From *Natrix natrix* L.

H. feideri Fain: From *N. natrix helvetica* Lac.

H. caheni Fain: From *Bitis nasicornis* Shaw and *Naja melanoleuca* Hall.

H. piger Berlese: From *Coluber gemonensis* Laur., *Elaphe situla* L., *N. natrix* L.

H. imphalensis Radford: From *Coluber radiatus* Schlegel.

H. novae-guineae Fain: From *Dendrophis calligaster salmonis* Gthr.

H. ophidius Lavoipierre: From *Causus lichtensteini* Jan.

H. schoutedeni Fain: From *Boaedon fuliginosus* Boie.

H. upembae Fain: From *Boaedon fuliginosus* Boie.

Asiatolaelaps tanneri Tibbetts: From *Natrix tigrina lateralis* Berth.

A. evansi Fain: From *Elaphe flavolineata* Schl.

Strandtibbettsia gordoni Tibbetts: From *Natrix* spp.

S. brasiliensis Fain: From *Lycognathus cervinus* Laur.

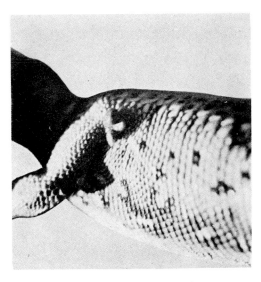

Fig. 354. *Lacerta agilis*. Leg infested by ticks. (Photo.: Stemmler-Gyger.)

Paramegistidae

Ophiomegistus luzonensis Banks: From snakes of Pacific islands.
O. buloloensis Gthr.: From snakes of Pacific islands.
O. clelandi Womersley: From Australian snakes.

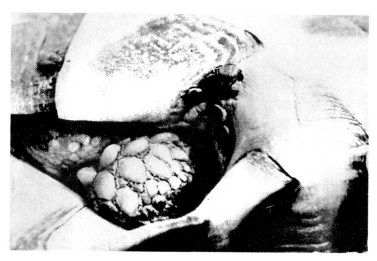

FIG. 355. *Testudo marginata.* Leg infested by ticks. (Photo.: Stemmler-Gyger.)

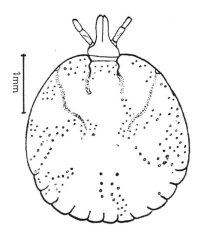

FIG. 356. *Amblyomma laticauda* Warburton (♂ of *Laticauda colubrina* Schneider). (After Warburton.)

Ixodides

These ticks have commonly been found to parasitize reptiles, particularly tortoises (Figs. 355, 356), snakes and varanids. *Ixodes ricinus* L., which employs three hosts, may in the nymphal stage invade reptiles, the final host being a mammal (Jellison, 1933). The argasid *Ornithodorus talaje* Guérin-Ménéville must be regarded as particularly dangerous because it transmits diseases caused by spirochaetes like Q-fever and others and may also infest humans. *Haemofilaria* may equally be transmitted by this tick.

Argasidae

Ornithodoros talaje Guérin-Ménéville.

Ixodidae

Numerous species of the genera *Amblyomma* (Fig. 356), *Aponomma* (Fig. 357) and *Hyalomma* as well as *Ixodes ricinus* L. have been found

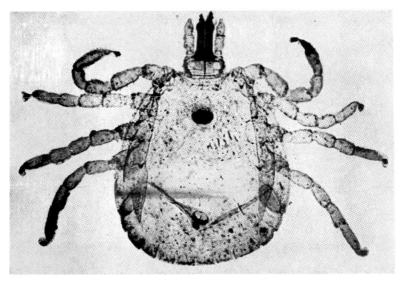

FIG. 357. *Aponomma latum* Koch. (Photo.: E. Elkan.)

on reptiles, particularly on tortoises, varanids and the larger snakes (Schulze, 1932, 1936; Dunn, 1918; Sambon, 1928; Krijgsman and Ponto, 1932; Warburton, 1932).

Trombidiformes

Pterygosomidae

We owe most of our knowledge on this family to R. F. Lawrence who reviewed it in 1935/36. He described mites infesting geckonids, agamids, gherrhosaurids and zonurids. On geckos he found:

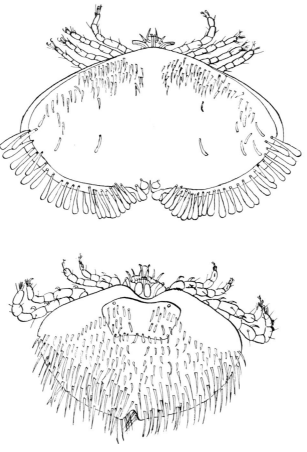

FIG. 358. Above: *Pterygosoma bedfordi* Lawr. Below: *Geckobia hemidactyli* Lawr.

Geckobia transvaalensis, G. ozambica, G. tasmani, G. oedurae, G. natalensis, G. hewitti, G. homopholus, G. namaquensis, G. rhoptropi, G. pachydactyli, G. hemidactyli (Fig. 358, below), *G. phyllodactyli*, and *G. karroica*.

The genus *Geckobia* was revised by Radford (1943). For further details see Hirst (1926) and Womersley (1941). They mention the following species:

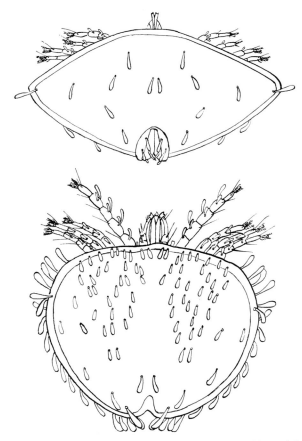

FIG. 359. Above: *Scaphothrix convexa* Lawr. Below: *Zonurobia cordylensis* Lawr.

Geckobia australis Hirst, *G. bataviensis* Vitzthum, *G. boulengeri* Hirst.
G. clelandi Hirst, *G. diversipilis* Hirst, *G. gehyrae* Hirst, *G. gleadoviana* Hirst.
G. gymnodactyli Womersley, *G. haplodactyli* Womersley, *G. hindustanica* Hirst.
G. indica Hirst, *G. latasti* Hirst, *G. loricata* Berlese, *G. papuana* Hirst.

G. malayana Hirst, *G. naultina* Womersley, *G. neumanni* Berlese, *G. similis* Tragardh.

G. socotrensis Hirst, *G. tarantulae* Tragardh.

G. turkestana Hirst.

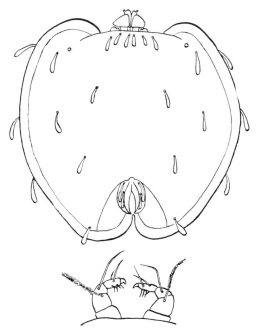

Fig. 360. *Ixodiderma inverta* (legs not shown). Below: palps. (From Lawrence.)

Of the genus *Pterygosoma* they mention:

Pterygosoma inermis Tragardh, *P. neumanni* Berlese and *P. persicum* Hirst.

From S. African agamids Lawrence (1935/6) mentions:

Pterygosoma melanum Hirst.

P. agamae Peters and the new species *P. hirsti, P. armatum, P. bedfordi* (Fig. 358, above).

P. longipalpe, P. aculeatum, P. triangulare and *P. transvaalense.*

From Gherrosaurids he quotes:

Pterygosoma gherrosauri Lawr., *P. bicolor* Lawr. and *P. hystrix* Lawr. The genera of this family were found on zonurids, particularly *Zonurobia* species newly described as: *Zonurobia cordylensis* (Fig. 359, bottom), *Z. polyzonensis, Z. circularis, Z. semilunaris, Z. debilipes, Z. transvaalensis, Z. sanguinea, Z. subquadrata* and *Z. montana.*

To these should be added:
Scaphothriz convexa Lawr. (Fig. 359, top).
Ixodiderma inverta Lawr. (Fig. 360), *I. lacertae* Lawr., *I. pilosa* Lawr.
Other authors described: *Pimeliaphilus insignis* Berlese, *P. tenuipes* Hirst, also occurring on geckonids.

Lane (1954), gave a detailed account of *Geckobiella texana* Banks found to infest *Sceloporus u. undulatus* Latr. (Fig. 361).

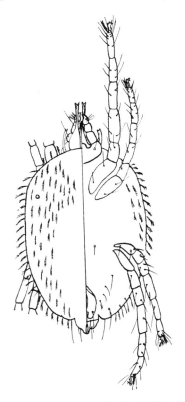

Fig. 361. *Geckobiella texana* Banks ♂. (From Lane.)

The following key for these species was given by Lawrence (1936):

1 With dorsal shield   2
  Without dorsal shield   3
2 Dorsal shield with a few, long hairs   *Pimeliaphilus*
  Dorsal shield with many but short hairs   *Geckobia*
3 Apex of hypostome broad, dorsal shield with few
    hairs   4

Hypostome nearly parallel, dorsal shield with
  many hairs   5
4 Body longer than wide, large, skin leathery   *Ixodiderma*
  Body wider than long, small, skin not leathery   *Scaphothrix*
5 Back with a group of hairs on either side of mouth
  organs. Eyeless   *Pterygosoma*
  Back without group of hairs around mouth, eyes
  present   *Zonurobia*

Trombiculidae

Like so many other animals reptiles are frequently infested by
chigger mites. These mites infest mammals as well as cold-blooded
animals: they do not seem to be very particular about their hosts and
the list given below may be incomplete. It rests mainly on the reviews
by Audy (1961), Lawrence (1949) and Radford (1942a). All these
species are ectoparasitic. There have been recorded:

Trombicula agamae André: From saurians.

T. *arenicola* Loomis: From *Masticophis flagellum* Shaw and *Phyllo-rhynchus decurtatus* Cope.

T. *hakei* Radford: From *Coluber radiatus* Schlegel and *Naja tripudians fasciatus* Gray.

T. *hasei* Feider: From Rumanian lizards.

T. *vanommereni* Schierbeck : From humans and saurians (Radford).

T. (*Eutrombicula*) *tropica* Ewing: From *Anaidia bitaeniata* Blg.-Venezuela.

T. (*Eu.*) *alfreddugesi* Oudemanns: Infests chelonians, snakes, lizards and birds. In the U.S.A. it causes dermatitis in humans. In E. Asia it transmits the Tsutsugamushi disease (Ewing, 1944).

T. (*Eu.*) *belkini* Gould: From Californian lizards—*Phrynosoma coronatum* Gray and *Uta stansburiana* Baird and Girard.

T. (*Eu.*) *gurneyi* Ewing: From *Eumeces fasciatus* L.

T. (*Eu.*) *insularis* Ewing: From *Anolis cybotes* Cope.

T. (*Eu.*) *ophidica* Fonseca: From *Ophis merremi* Wagler.

T. (*Eu.*) *tinami* Oudemans: From *Crypturus noctivagus* Wied.

T. (*Eutrombicula, Squamicola* Lawrence) *draconis* Lawr.: From *Pseudocordylus s. subviridis.*

T. (*Eu. Squ.*) *lawrenci* Wharton and Fuller: From agamids.

T. (*Eu. Squ.*) *montensis* Lawr.: From *Pseudocordylus s. subviridis.*

Lawrence (1949) furthermore described the following species from
saurians:

T. (*Eu. Squ.*) *gherrosauri, T. homopholis, T. pachydactyli, T. rhodes-iensis, T. rhoptropi.*

T. (Fonseca) ewingi Fonseca: From *Ophis merremi*, Wagler.

T. (F.) travassosi Fonseca: From *Spilotes pullatus* L.

T. (Neotrombicula) tragardhiana Feider: From *Lacerta agilis* L.

Acomatacarus arizonensis Ewing: From *Phrynosoma coronatum blainvillei* Gray, *Sceloporus m. magister* Hallowell and other saurians.

Other species, found by Lawrence to infest saurians, are:

A. geckobius, A. lacertae, A. mabuyae, A. namaquensis.

Ascoschöngastia gherrosauri Lawr., *A. ophicola* Lawr., *A. tropidosauri* Lawr., *A. viperina* Lawr.

Euschöngastia lacertae Brennan: From *Sceloporus occidentalis* Baird and Girard, and *Gherronotus multicarinatus* Blainville.

Eu. longitarsala Powder and Loomis: From *Uta stansburiana* Baird and Girard, *Phrynosoma coronatum* Gray, *Phrynosoma platyrhinos* and other Californian lizards.

Neoschöngastia scelopori Ewing: From *Sceloporus spinosus* Wiegm.

Odontacarus australis Ewing: From *Tropidurus peruvianus* Lesson.

O. shawi Brennan: From *Gecko coleonyx variegatus* Baird, *Masticophis flagellum* Shaw and other Californian lizards and snakes.

Sauracarella africana Lawr., *S. montana* Lawr., *S. whartoni* Lawr.

Sauriscus ewingi Lawr.

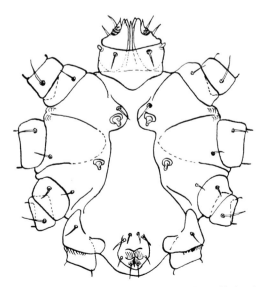

Fig. 362. *Ophioptes tropicalis* Ewing. (From Ewing.)

Schöngastia mabuyana Lawr., *Sch. platysauri* Lawr., *Sch. pseudo-cordyli* Lawr.

Sch. scincicola Lawr.

For details the original papers should be consulted.

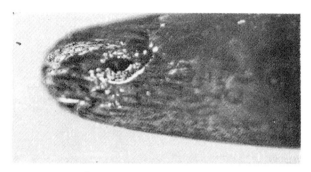

FIG. 363. *Anguis fragilis* ♀. Eye region infested with the hypopus stage of the tick *Caloglyphus*. (Photo.: E. Elkan.)

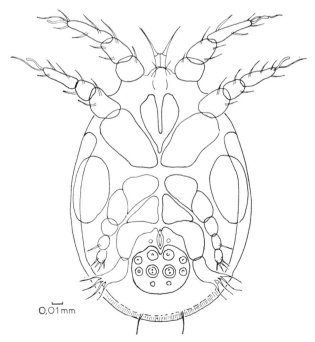

0,01mm

FIG. 364. Hypopus stage of the tick *Caloglyphus*. Drawn by microprojection. (E. Elkan.)

Myobiidae

This is a small group of mites which live on the scales of S. American snakes. *Ophioptes parkeri* Sambon, *O. tropicalis* Ewing (Fig. 362), *O. oudemansi* Sambon.

Erythraeidae

Species of the genus *Leptus*, occurring on lizards inhabiting Pacific islands were described by Baker and Wharton (1952).

Sarcoptiformes

One of us (E. Elkan) had occasion to observe the infestation of a slow-worm (*Anguis fragilis* L.) with numerous specimens of the hypopus stage of a *Caloglyphus* species. Since, at the hypopus stage, these juvenile mites have no functional mouth organs, they were apparently using the slow-worm as an intermediate transport host and the case cannot be regarded as one of true parasitism (Figs. 363, 364).

REFERENCES

André, M. (1929). Nouvelle forme larvaire de *Thrombicula*, parasite sur un saurien de Palestine. *Bull. Mus. Nat. Hist. Nat.* 401–405.

Audy, J. R. (1961). African *Trombiculidae* (*Acarina*). 2. The genera *Eutrombicula* Ew. and *Sauriscus* Lawr. with description of a new subgenus, *Squamicola*. *Ann. Natal. Mus.* **15**, 135–140.

Baker, E. W. and Wharton, G. W. (1925). "An Introduction to Acarology." New York.

Camin, J. H. (1948). Mite transmission of a haemorrhagic septicaemia in snakes. *J. Parasit.* **34**, 545–554.

Camin, J. H. (1953). Observations on the life history and sensory behaviour of the snake mite. (*Ophionyssus natricis* Gervais) (Acarina, Macronyssidae). *Chicago Acad. Sci. Publ.* 10.

Dunn, L. H. (1918). Studies on the Iguana tick *Amblyomma dissimilis* in Panama. *J. Parasit.* **5**, 1–10.

Ewing, H. E. (1934). A new pit-producing mite from the scales of a S. American snake. *Parasitology* **20**, 53–56.

Ewing, H. E. (1944). The trombiculid mites (Chigger mites) and their relation to disease. *J. Parasit.* **30**, 339–365.

Fain, A. (1961). Les Acariens parasites endopulmonaires des serpents (*Entonyssidae Mesostigmata*). *Bull. Inst. Roy. Soc. Nat. Belg.* **37**, 1–135.

Fain, A. (1961b). Espèces et genres nouveaux dans la famille *Ixodorhynchidae* Ewing 1922 (*Acarina: Mesostigmata*). *Rev. Zool. Bot. Afr.* **64**, 175–182.

Fain, A. (1961c). Une nouvelle famille d'Acariens, parasite de serpents du genre *Mehelya* au Congo: *Omentolaelaptidae* fam. nov. (Mesostigmata). *Rev. Zool. Bot. Afr.* **64**, 283–296.

Fain, A. (1962). Les Acariens mesostigmatiques ectoparasites des Serpents. *Bull. Inst. R. Sci. Nat. Belg.* **38**, 18, 1–149.

Feider, Z. (1958). Sur une larve du genre *Trombicula* (*Acari*) parasite sur les lézards de la Roumanie. *Z. Parasitenk.* **18**, 441–456.

Finnegan, S. (1931). On a new species of mite of the family Heterozerconidae, parasitic on a snake. *Proc. zool. Soc. Lond.*, 1349–1357.

Fonseca, F. da, (1934). Der Schlangenparasit *Ixobioides butantanensis* novi generis n. sp. (*Acarina, Ixodorhynchidae*, nov. fam.). *Z. Pa asitenk.* **6**, 508–527.

Fonseca, F. da (1948). A monograph of the genera and species of *Macronyssidae* Oudemans 1936, (syn. *Liponyssidae* Vitzthum 1931 Acari). *Proc. zool. Soc. Lond.* **118**, 249–334.

Hirst, S. (1915). On a blood-sucking gamasid mite (*Ichoronyssus serpentinus* sp. n?) parasitic on Couper's snake. *Proc. zool. Soc. Lond.*, 383–386.

Hirst, S. (1926). On the parasitic mites of the suborder *Prostigmata* (*Trombidioidea*) found on lizards. *J. Linn. Soc. Zool.* **36**, 173–200.

Jellison, W. L. (1933). The parasitism of Lizards by *Ixodes ricinus californicus*. *J. Parasit.* **20**, 243–244.

Johnston, D. (1962). Ixodorhynchine mites ectoparasites of snakes. 1. Descriptions of a new genus and three new species from the nearctic region. (Acarina Mesostigmata). *Bull. Ann. Soc. R. Ent. Belg.* **98**, Nr. 11.

Krijgsman, B. J. and Ponto, S. A. S. (1932). Die Verbreitung der Zecken in Niederländisch-Ostindien. *Z. Parasitenk.* **4**, 140–146.

Lane, J. E. (1954). A redescription of the American lizard mite *Geckobiella texana* Banks 1904 with notes on the systematics of the species. (*Acarina: Pterygosomidae*). *J. Parasit.* **40**, 93–99.

Lawrence, R. F. (1935). Prostigmatic mites of S. African lizards. *Parasitology* **27**, 1–45.

Lawrence, R. F. (1936). The prostigmatic mites of S. African lizards. *Parasitology* **28**, 1–39.

Lawrence, R. F. (1949). The larval trombiculid mites of S. African vertebrates. *Ann. Natal. Mus.* **11**, 405–486.

Powder, W. A. and Loomis, R. B. (1962). A new species and new records of Chiggers (*Acarina: Trombiculidae*) from reptiles of S. California. *J.Parasit.* **48**, 204–208.

Privora, M. and Samsinak, K. (1958). Milben als Menschenplage. *Z. Parasitenk.* **18**, 257–269.

Radford, C. D. (1942a). The larval Trombiculinae (Acarina: Trombidiinae) with descriptions of twelve new species. *Parasitology* **34**, 55–81.

Radford, C. D. (1942b). New parasitic mites (*Acarina*). *Parasitology* **34**, 295–307.

Radford, C. D. (1943). Genera and species of parasitic mites (*Acarina*). *Parasitology* **35**, 58–81.

Sambon, L. W. (1928). The parasitic acarians of animals and the part they play in the causation of the eruptive fevers and other diseases of man. *Ann. trop. Med. Parasit.* **22**, 67–132.

Schmidt, F. L. (1928). *Entonyssus vitzthumi* (Acarina), a new ophidian lung mite. *J. Parasit.* **26**, 309–313.

Schroeder, C. R. (1934). Snake mite (*Ophionyssus serpentinum*). *J. Econ. Ent.* **27**, 1004–1014.

Schulze, P. (1932). Neue und wenig bekannte Arten der Zeckengattungen *Amblyomma* und *Aponomma*. *Z. Parasitenk.* **4**, 459–476.

Schulze, P. (1936). Neue und wenig bekannte Amblyommen und Aponommen aus Afrika, Südamerika, Indien, Borneo und Australien. (*Ixodidae*). *Z. Parasitenk.* **8**, 419–637.

Schweizer, H. (1952). Die Blutmilbe (*Ophionyssus natricis* Gerv./Mégn.) der "Stallfeind" des Schlangenpflegers und ihre Vernichtung. *Aqu. Terr. Z.* **5**, 103–105.

Strandtmann, R. W. and Wharton, G. W. (1958). "A Manual of Mesostigmatic Mites Parasitic on Vertebrates." Maryland.

Till, W. M. (1957). Mesostigmatic mites, living as parasites of reptiles in the Ethiopian region (*Acarina: Laelaptidae*). *J. Ent. Soc. S. Afr.* **20** (1) 120–143.

Warburton, C. (1932). On five new species of ticks (*Arachnida: Ixodidae*). *Parasitology* **24**, 558–568.

Womersley, H. (1941). New species of *Geckobia* (*Acarina: Pterygosomidae*) from Australia and New Zealand. *Trans. Roy. Soc. S. Austr.* **65**, 323–328.

J. Tongue Worms (Linguatulida)

These parasites, which are not worms but related to the Arachnida, may be found infesting tropical snakes and saurians. Fain (1961) found 11% of fifty-two examined specimens of *Naja* in the National Parks of Albert and Gramba (Belgian Congo) infected with *Cubirea pomeroyi* Woodl. Sixteen specimen of the genus *Mehelya* from the same area were parasitized by *Porocephalus subulifer* Leuckart. An infection with two different species of tongue worms was found in two cases only. In general the infections seem to exclude each other.

Most linguatulids are entoparasites and live, in reptiles, in the bronchi, the lungs, rarely in the heart or in the head. Only in a few cases has it been possible to determine their life cycle. Most of them seem to require two hosts. Reptiles become infected by feeding on primary hosts containing juvenile stages. These may be fish, amphibians, reptiles and mammals, rarely birds. Some species seem to complete their whole development without change of host. In such a case larvae and adults are found side by side. This, as Fain (1961) points out, is however no final proof, since the larvae need not have developed in the same host but may have been taken up with infected food. The presence of very young stages between the embryo and the third larva might be more suggestive (Fig. 372). Fain and Mortelmans (1960) found, in the trachea of a Komodo dragon, a female with mature ĕggs as well as encysted second and later larvae of *Sambonia lohrmanni* Noc and Giglioni, and considered this as sufficient proof for continuous development in one and the same host. But it may happen that linguatulid larvae re-encyst on entry into a new host before attaining sexual maturity. Fain (1961), whose original papers should be consulted for the determination of species, distinguished fifty different types of Linguatulida, as follows:

Order Cephalobaenida

Cephalobaenidae

Pulmonary parasites.

Cephalobaena tetrapoda Heymons: In S. American snakes of the genera *Bothrops, Lachesis, Leptophis* (Fig. 365a).

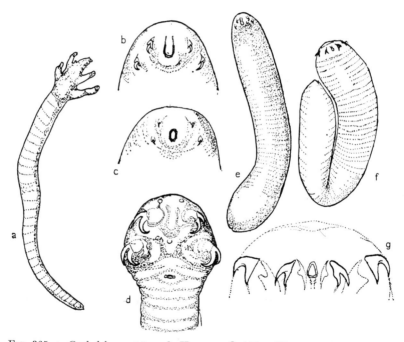

Fig. 365. a, *Cephalobaena tetrapoda* Heymons ♀. (After Heymons.) b, and e, *Alofia platycephala* Giglioli ♀. (After Heymons.) c, *Sebekia oxycephala* Sambon ♀. (After Heymons.) d, *Leiperia gracilis* Heymons and Vitzthum. Head of immature worm. (From Heymons.) f, *Elenia lialisi* Heymons second larval stage. (After Heymons.) g, Head of *Elenia lialisi* Heymons.

Raillietiella geckonis Sambon: Adult in geckonids and agamids.

R. affinis Bovien: In *Gecko verticillatus* Laur.

R. mabuiae Heymons: In *Mabuya sulcata* Peters (Fig. 366, left).

R. gehyrae Bovien: In *Gehyra multilata* Wiegm.

R. hemidactyli Hett.: In S.E. Asian geckonids.

R. kochi Heymons: In varanids.

R. shipleyi Heymons: In varanids.

R. orientalis Sambon: Adult in Eurasian snakes, larval in a species of *Naja* from the Congo.

R. boulengeri Sambon (Fig. 366, middle and right): larval and adult in African snakes.

R. agcoi Tubangui and Masilungan: In Philippine cobras.

R. mediterranea Sambon: Larval in toads, adult in *Coluber* spp.

R. furcocerca Sambon: In S. American snakes.

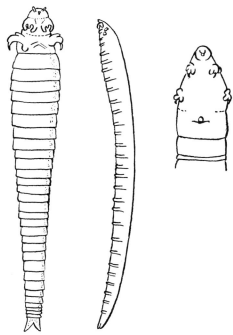

FIG. 366. Left, *Raillietiella mabuiae* Heymons. Middle and right, *Raillietiella boulengeri* Vaney and Sambon. (From Kükenthal, 1926.)

R. bicaudata Heymons and Vitzthum: In N. American snakes.

R. giglioli Hett: In *Amphisbaena alba* L.

R. chamaeleonis Gretillat and Brygoo: In Chamaeleonids.

R. schoutedeni Fain: In *Monopeltis schoutedeni* Witte (Fig. 367).

Megadrepanoides solomonensis Self and Kunz: In the lungs of *Varanus indicus* Daud.

M. varani Self and Kunz: In the lungs of *Varanus indicus* Daudin.

Order Porocephalida

Sebekidae

Sebekia oxycephala Sambon: in the lungs of American crocodiles (adult). Larval in American fish and snakes (Fig. 365c).

S. wedli Gigliolo: Adult in African crocodiles.
S. acuminata Travassos: In Brazilian crocodiles.
S. divesta Giglioli: In American crocodiles.

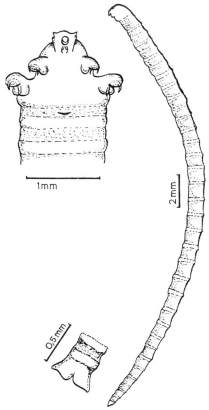

FIG. 367. *Raillietiella schoutedeni* Fain. (After Fain.)

S. samboni Travassos: In Brazilian crocodiles.
S. cesarisi Giglioli: In African crocodiles.
S. jubini Sambon: In the nasal pit of *Crocodilus siamensis* Sch.
Diesingia megastoma Diesing: In *Hydraspis geoffroyana* Wagler.
Alofia platycephala Giglioli: In S. American crocodiles (Fig. 365b, e).
A. indica Hett: In crocodiles from the Ganges.
Leiperia gracilis Heymans and Vitzthum: Adult in S. American croco-
diles, larval in fish, turtles and snakes (= *Pentastomum gracile*
Diesing) (Fig. 365d).

L. cincinnalis Sambon: Adult in lungs, heart and aorta of *Crocodilus niloticus* Laur. Larval in several spp. of fish (= *Porocephalus nematoides* de Beauchamp) (Fig. 372b).

Subtriquetridae

Adult in the oral cavity and the pharynx of crocodiles, larval in the intestine and swim-bladder of fish.

Subtriquetra subtriquetra Sambon: In S. American crocodiles.

S. shipleyi Hett: In the pharynx of Indian crocodiles.

S. megacephala Sambon: In the cephalic tissues of *Crocodilus palustris* L.

Sambonidae

Sambonia lohrmanni Noc and Giglioli: Larval and adult in the lungs of African varanids (Fig. 368).

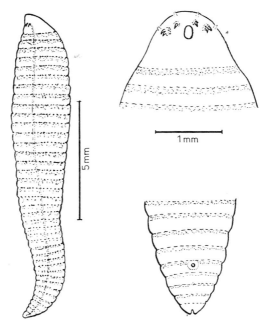

FIG. 368. *Sambonia lohrmanni* Noc and Giglioli. (After Fain and Mortelmans.)

Elenia australis Heymons: In Australian varanids.

E. lialisi Heymons: Larval in *Lialis jicari* Blgr. (Fig. 365f.).

Waddycephalus teretiusculus Sambon: Larval and adult in Australian snakes (Fig. 369a).

Porocephalidae

Larval in mammals, adult in the lungs of snakes.

Porocephalus crotali Humboldt: Larval in mammals (mice), snakes and amphibians. Adult in crotalid snakes.

P. clavatus Sambon: Larvae encysted in mammals; adult in boid and viperid snakes.

P. stilesi Sambon: In S. American snakes.

P. subulifer Sambon: Larval in snakes and mammals, adult in African snakes (Fig. 370, right).

P. benoiti Fain: In African snakes.

P. pomeroyi Woodland: In African snakes.

Kiricephalus coarctatus Sambon: In American snakes, larval encysted in snakes and mammals (Fig. 369b).

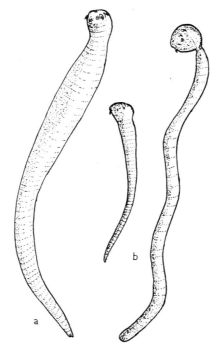

FIG. 369. a, *Waddycephalus teretiusculus* Sambon ♀; b, *Kiricephalus coarctatus* Sambon: left, ♂; right, ♀. (After Heymons.)

K. pattoni Sambon: Larval in snakes and amphibians, adult in Indian, Madagascar and Australian snakes.

K. tortus Sambon: In *Dipsadomorphus irregularis* Merrem.

Armilliferidae

Nymphs mostly in mammals, rarely in birds, adult in the lungs of snakes.

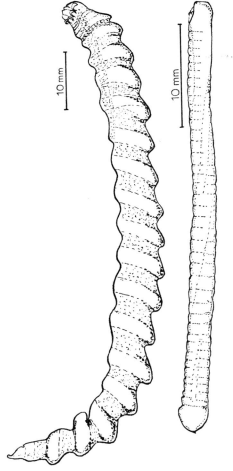

Fig. 370. Left, *Armillifer armillatus* Wyman; right, *Porocephalus subulifer* Leuckart. (After Fain.)

Armillifer armillatus Sambon (Figs. 370, left; 371, right). In boid, viperid and colubrid snakes, larval in mammals including humans, rarely in birds.

A. grandis Sambon: Larval in birds. Adult in African viperid snakes.

A. moniliformis Sambon: Larval in monkeys, tarsians and carnivores. Adult in Asian pythons.

Cubirea annulata Kishida: In African snakes.

C. pomeroyi Kishida: In *Naja* spp.

Gigliolella brumpti Chabaud and Choquet: In snakes from Madagascar.

Ligamifer mazzai Heymons: In Asian and Australian snakes. Perhaps transmitted by marsupials.

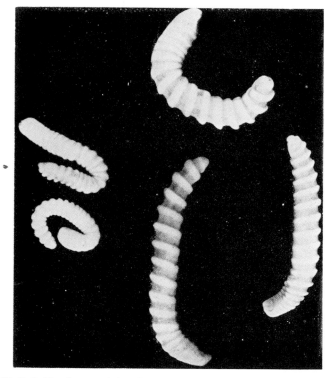

Fig. 371. Left, Two larvae of *Armillifer grandis* Hett; right, three larvae of *Armillifer armillatus* Wyman. (After Fain.)

REFERENCES

Fain, A. (1961). Les Pentastomides de l'Afrique Centrale. *Ann. Koninkl. Mus. Tervuren* **92**, 1–115.

Fain, A. and Mortelmans, J. (1960). Observations sur le cycle évolutif de *Sambonia lohrmanni* chez le Varan. Preuve d'un dévelopement direct chez les Pentastomida. *Bull. Acad. Roy. Belg.* 5. ser. **46**, 518–531.

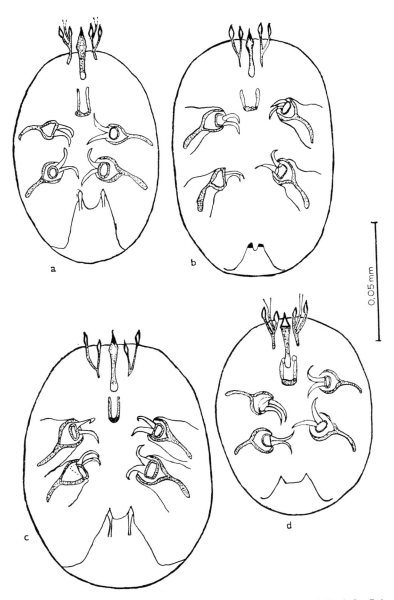

Fig. 372. a, Embryonic stage of *Sambonia lohrmanni* Noc and Giglioni; b, *Leiperia cincinnalis* Sambon; c, *Armillifer armillatus* Wyman; d, *Porocephalus subulifer* Leuckart. (After Fain.)

Gretillat, S. and Brygoo (1959). *Raillietiella chamaeleonis* n. sp. première espèce de *Cephalobaenidae* (*Pentastomida*) signalée à Madagascar. *Ann. Parasit.* **34**, 112–120.

Hett, M. L. (1924). On the family *Linguatulidae*. *Proc. zool. Soc. Lond.* 107–160.

Heymons, R. (1932). Ein Beitrag zur Kenntnis der Pentastomiden Australiens und benachbarter Gebiete. *Z. Parasitenk.* **4**, 409–430.

Heymons, R. (1935). Beiträge zur Systematik der Pentastomiden. II. Einige bemerkenswerte Pentastomiden aus Lacertiliern. *Z. Parasitenk.* **10**, 676–690.

Heymons, R. and Graf Vitzthum, H. (1935). Beiträge zur Systematik der Pentastomiden. *Z. Parasitenk.* **8**, 1–103.

Self, J. P. and Murry, F. S. (1948). *Porocephalus crotali* Humboldt (Pentastomida) in Oklahoma. *J. Parasit.* **34**, 21–23.

Woodland, W. N. F. (1920). On a remarkable new species of *Porocephalus* (*P. pomeroyi* sp. n.) from the foregut of a Nigerian cobra. *Parasitology* **12**, 337–340.

K. INSECTS

Insects may damage Reptilia directly and indirectly; directly through stinging and blood-sucking and through the proteolytic action of fly larvae. Peters (1948) and Rainey (1953) reported on cases of this kind in chelonians. Equally Graham-Jones (1961) mentions that flies frequently deposit their eggs in the cloacal and tail region of chelonians. The larvae, when hatched, penetrate the host tissue and may cause deep wounds extending under the carapace. Any visible larvae should be removed. The tortoises should be bathed twice daily and treated with antiseptic powder. If not too heavily damaged the animals may be saved.

Indirect insect damage to reptiles may be caused by mosquitoes and flies which transmit blood parasites. The following might be mentioned:

Culex fatigans Wied
C. annulirostis Skuse } transmit filariae.

Culex tarsalis L.   transmits viruses.

Phlebotomus spp.   transmit *Bartonella* spp., *Leishmania* spp. and trypanosomes.

Glossina palpalis Rob. and Desv.
G. tachinoides Westwood } transmit trypanosomes.

In a few cases even fleas have been found on reptiles. Jäth (1952) encountered these insects on *Lacerta vivipara* Jacquin and on *Natrix natrix* L. Fleas have also been found on the green lizard *Lacerta v. viridis* Laur. which had hatched from the faeces of dogs and were determined as *Ctenocephalus canis* L. (T. Schellkopf in Jäth, 1952).

We may finally mention *Triatoma rubrovaria* Pinto, a bug which has been found to carry spores of the protozoon *Hepatozoon triatomae*

Osimani which is a parasite of lizards. The bugs, most probably, transmit the infection.

REFERENCES

Graham-Jones, O. (1961). Notes on the common tortoise, *Vet. Rec.* **73**, 313–321.
Jäth, H. (1952). Flöhe als Irrgäste auf Reptilien. *Aqu. Terr. Z.* **5**, 276.
Peters, J. A. (1948). The box turtle as a host for dipterous parasites. *Amer. Midl. Nat.* **40**, 472–474.
Rainey, D. G. (1953). Death of an ornate box turtle parasitized by dipterous larvae. *Herpetologica* **9**, 109–110.

L. DISEASES CAUSED BY FUNGI

Contrary to our findings in fish and amphibians mycotic diseases in reptiles are rare. We quote the few accounts of such infections which have been published.

Meyn (1942) described the appearance of *Actinomyces bovis* Harz em. Boström in a captive snake. Equally Rodhain and Mattlet (1950) found fungal threads in a tracheal tumour of a snake. From these a *Cephalosporium* type fungus could be grown in culture.

Blanchard (1890) found various stages of a hypomycetous fungus in tumours of a green lizard (*Lacerta viridis* L.). Both the surface layers and the deeper parts of the tumours contained whitish conidia, divided into chambers and having a length of up to 15 μ. The deeper layers showed a dense network of chambered, laterally compressed threads resembling *Fusarium* or *Selenosporium*. Species of the former genus may be found on animal corpses. The fungus also had great similarity to *Selenosporium urticum*, a species which grows on decaying plants, and the author suggests that it may have been identical with the latter species.

One of us (E. E.) saw a mycotic infection in a specimen of *Coronella austriaca* kept in company with a specimen of *Natrix sipedon*. The latter died first, showing no other sign of illness than a small swelling under one scale. A month after this the smooth snake showed signs of disease. The nostrils were blocked, the oral mucosa swollen, one eye more prominent than the other and the whole gular region oedematous. The oedema disappeared after the snake had been killed. Post-mortem examination revealed numerous white spots on the liver (Fig. 373). These contained no acid-fast bacilli but many hyphenous fungal threads. Attempts to grow bacteria from any part of the snake failed. The fungal threads were Gram-positive and stained well by the periodic acid–Schiff technique. The peripheral part of the foci and the surrounding tissue contained large numbers of eosinophil granulocytes.

Fungal mycelia were also found (E. E.) on the peritoneal surface of abdominal organs in a specimen of *Chinemys reevesii* Gray which had suffered from an extensive disease of the Harderian gland (Fig. 374). It was not possible to determine the exact nature of these fungi.

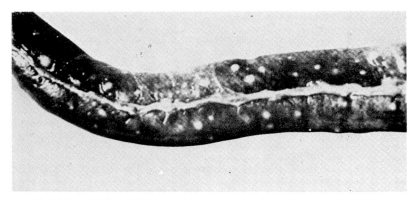

FIG. 373. Liver of *Coronella a. austriaca* with multiple fungal abscesses. × 4. (Photo.: E. Elkan.)

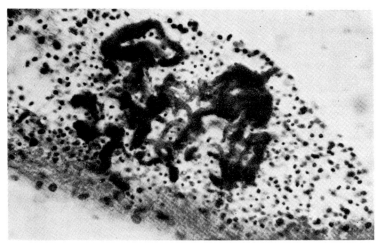

FIG. 374. Fungal mycelium in the peritoneal cavity of *Chinemys reevesii* Gray in a specimen also suffering from a diseased Harderian gland. × 250. (Photo.: E. Elkan.)

Some authors consider that fungi may be responsible for an oral disease of tortoises, sometimes described as mouth cancer (Graham-Jones, 1961).

Interesting observations on zoophagous fungi were published by Hunt (1957). He found that the lungs of tortoises were frequently the seat of fungi of an *Aspergillus* type. In severe cases such an infection may entirely destroy and obliterate parts of the organ. Confinement of several animals in close quarters increases the danger of transmission. The author concluded that about 3% of all deaths in captive tortoises were caused by pulmonary mycosis.

Fungal infection may even extend to the carapace of tortoises. Infection by *Mucor* species has been observed in such cases but the exact pathogens have not been determined. The ventral shield is more frequently affected than the dorsal carapace. All types of chelonians may be so affected with the exception of marine species, where the disease is much rarer. A species very commonly affected is *Sternotherus carinatus* Gray.

Four specimens of giant tortoises (*Testudo elephantopus, T. gigantea elephantina*) died in the Chicago Zoological Park (Georg et al., 1962). The first showed a lung infection with *Aspergillus amstelodami* and *Geotrichum candidum*. The second, also a Galapagos tortoise, was infected with *Beauveria bassiana*, the third, an aldabra tortoise, with *Paecilomyces fumoso-roseus*, in the fourth no certain cause of death was ascertained. The two Galapagos tortoises had been in captivity for 30 years. The authors stress the difficulty in imitating the exact environmental conditions to which these giant tortoises are geared. Their particular temperature requirements cannot always be maintained and they may become victims of bacterial and fungal infections against which they have no natural immunity.

Among the reptiles most difficult to keep in captivity are the chameleons. In spite of all our efforts most of them die within a year and the exact cause of death usually remains unexplained. We were therefore particularly interested in the case of a two-banded chameleon (*Chamaeleo bitaeniatus* Fischer 1884) which, as related by its owner, had developed a "paraplegia" and had to be killed because it could no longer maintain its hold on branches and fell to the ground unless helped. The dissection of *Chamaeleo bitaeniatus* is difficult because the entire peritoneum is intensely black through the presence of innumerable melanophores. The fact that this chameleon died from an extensive disease of the liver was therefore only discovered when sections of this organ were examined (Fig. 375a). These showed the liver permeated by foci of necrotic material surrounded first by a shell of granulation tissue and then by a second shell of fibrous tissue. Application of the periodic acid–Schiff technique showed the granulation zone to be heavily permeated by a yeast-like fungus, the individual cells measuring between 2·5 ×3 μ to 7 ×8 μ. They showed no sign of capsule formation but some filamentation with branching and septation, the hyphae being between 1·5 and 2·0 μ thick. Dr. J. G. Murray of the Mycological

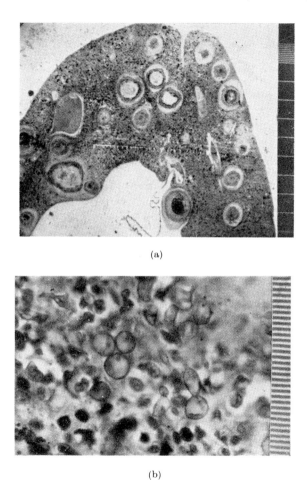

(a)

(b)

Fɪɢ. 375. *Chamaeleo bitaeniatus* Fischer. Adult female. Infection of liver with *Candida albicans*. (a) H. and E. Low power. Scale: 0·1 and 0·01. (b) PAS-haematoxylin-tetrazin. Scale 1·67 μ. (Photo.: E. Elkan.)

Reference Laboratory of the London School of Hygiene who examined the material considered the offending organism to be most likely *Candida albicans*. Considering how extensively the liver of this reptile was affected its death is perhaps not surprising. What seems more extraordinary is the fact that nothing abnormal and in particular no fungus could be found in any of the other viscera although a thorough search was made in microscopic sections. Further material of this kind would be of great interest particularly since we should like to know whether chameleons frequently die of fungal infections or whether this was an unusual and isolated case (Fig. 375b).

REFERENCES

Blanchard, R. (1890). Sur une remarquable dermatose causée chez le lézard vert par un champion du genre *Selenosporium. Mem. Soc. Zool. Fr.* **3**, 241–255.
Georg, L. K., Williamson, W. M., Tilden, E. B. and Getty, R. E. (1962). Mycotic pulmonary disease of captive giant tortoises due to *Beauveria bassiana* and *Poecilomyces fumoso-roseus. Sabouraudia* **2**, 80–86.
Graham-Jones, O. (1961). Notes on the Common Tortoise. *Vet. Rec.* **73**, 313–321.
Hunt, T. J. (1957). Notes on diseases and mortality in testudines. *Herpetologica* **13**, 19–23.
Meyn, A. (1942). Actinomyces Infektion bei einer Schlange. *Zool. Garten* N.F. **14**, 251.
Rodhain J. and Mattlet, G. (1950). Une tumeur mycosique chez la couleuvre vipérine *Tropidonotus natrix. Ann. Parasit.* **25**, 77–79

CHAPTER 21

Non-Parasitic and Environmental Diseases

A. TUMOURS

Like the fish and the Amphibia, reptiles may be afflicted by a variety of tumours which may be genuine or of the pseudotumour variety. The genuine tumours may be benign, causing displacement of neighbouring

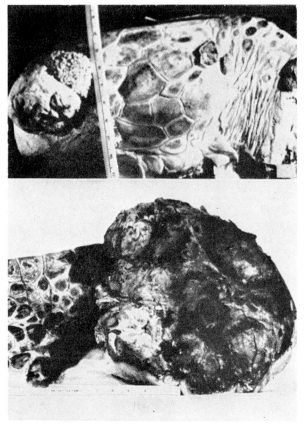

FIG. 376. Dermal papillomata in *Chelonia mydas* L. Above, tumour above the eye; below, tumour on the tail. (From Lucké and Schlumberger.)

organs only, or malign, infiltrating the neighbourhood and metastasizing. Lucké and Schlumberger (1949) reviewed the material available.

Dermal tumours (epitheliomata and papillomata) were described by Schwarz (1923) on *Tupinambis teguixin*; by Lucké and Schlumberger (1948) on *Pelusios odoratus* Latr.; and by Lucké, Smith and Coates (1938) on *Chelonia mydas* (Fig. 376). Smith and Coates suggest that the dermal fibroepitheliomata seen on the skin of marine turtles may have been caused by a virus because similar eruptions were seen on the skin of the indigenous human population. They also report the occasional presence of trematode eggs in these tumours.

Papillomata are commonly seen in the skin of lizards particularly in *Lacerta agilis* L. In its harmless form the disease is often referred to as "pox". Stolk and Plehn (1911) reported on such tumours in lizards which, in more extended form, may lead to the development of "tree bark tumours"; the histology of these was investigated by Klein (1952). The tumours may assume very bizarre shapes (Fig. 378) due to the development of a mixed fibroepithelial papilloma involving the epidermis and the corium. The cause of this disease, which has also been seen in freshly caught animals, is not known. Blanchard (1890) assigned responsibility to fungi of the *Selenosporium* type. Later authors could not confirm these findings. Papillary dermal carcinomata were seen by Bergmann (1941) in *Homalopsis buccata* L. and by Koch (1904) in *Lacerta agilis*. Similar observations were made by Pick and Poll (1903) and Plimmer (1912). Schlumberger (1958) published the figure of an epithelioma on the foot of *Heloderma*, the gila monster. In this case squamous epithelium had invaded the adjacent fibro-muscular tissue (Fig. 377) and even the underlying bone was affected.

One of us (E.E.) recently saw a very young chameleon (*Ch. bitaeniatus*) of 5 cm length whose mother had died of a liver infection by the fungus *Candida albicans*. Exactly the same fungus was seen growing in small patches on the skin of the youngster where it caused appreciable thickening of the stratum corneum and a thinning out of the layer of dermal melanophores. This picture seems to represent the typical reptilian reaction to any agent which chronically irritates the skin. Both fungi and viruses seem to be able occasionally to breach the epidermal defences in which case the disease progresses towards papillomatosis or even ulceration.

The oral tissue of reptiles is frequently affected by tumours. These were reviewed by Schlumberger (1953). At that time twenty cases had been reported from chelonians, crocodiles, lizards and snakes, not always arising from the same cause. Some of the tumours were multiple chondromata arising from cartilage, as for instance a tumour seen in a monitor lizard by Bland-Sutton (1885). The picture was also shown of a spongy carcinoma of the parotid in the Teju, *Tupinambis nigropunctatus* (Fig. 380).

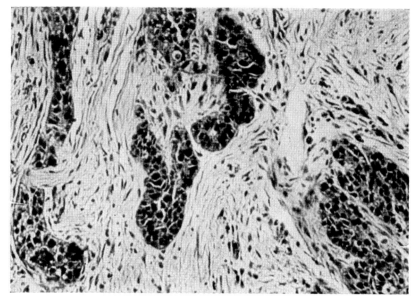

FIG. 377. Strands of a malign epithelioma invading the leg of a gila monster (*Heloderma suspectum*). × 220. (After Schlumberger in Cohrs, Jaffé and Meesen.)

Schlumberger mentions a pelvic tumour in a specimen of *Python reticulatus* from the Zoological Gardens of Philadelphia, accompanied by two melanomas elsewhere. We shall also have to report on a case of a melanosarcoma affecting the lip of a snake. Another oral tumour of a specimen of *Python sebae* Gm. was mentioned by Vaillant and Pettit (1902).

An ocular tumour in the turtle *Chelonia mydas* L. was seen by Lucké (1938).

We have already mentioned the occurrence of chondromata and osteomata in reptiles. Stolk (1958) for instance saw numerous small tumours in the tail of a *Lacerta viridis* L. and he could show that the tumour originated in the vertebral column. They contained osteoblasts, fibroblasts, bundles of collagen fibres and small fragments of bone. It was thought unlikely that the condition should have been the result of an injury. We may here also mention a case of bony tumours and malformation seen in a specimen of *Crocodilus porosus* Schneider by Kälin

(1937). Both exostoses and bony tumours were found in the same animal.

Tumours of internal organs have been found in the lungs (Bland-Sutton, 1885), the kidneys and the pancreas. A papillary adenocarcin-

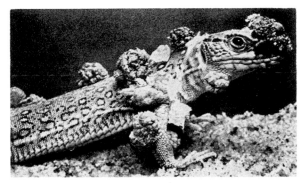

FIG. 378. *Lacerta ocellata* with tree bark tumours of the skin. (Photo.: Foersch.)

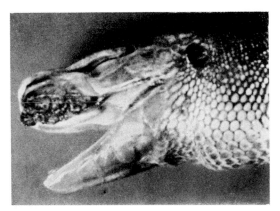

FIG. 379. Maxillary osteoma in *Lacerta viridis*. (Photo.: E. Elkan.)

oma of the kidney was seen by Patay (1933) in a specimen of *Natrix natrix* L. Ratcliffe (1935, 1943) described adenocarcinomata and other neoplasms of the pancreas.

Neural tumours are rare in reptiles. However, Scott and Beattie (1927) found a tumour of the cerebellum in *Crocodilus porosus* Schn.

Coloured tumours, particularly melanomata which occur in reptiles are rightly regarded with much apprehension. Ball (1946) reported on a remarkable case of melanoma in a specimen of *Pituophis melanoleucus*

Daudin. A melanoma appeared on the body of a female and on the lip of the male. The latter grew very rapidly to a size of 4×2.5 cm.

Pseudotumours, i.e. tumours due to parasitic infection, are frequently seen. To this group belong the gular tumours which were found to

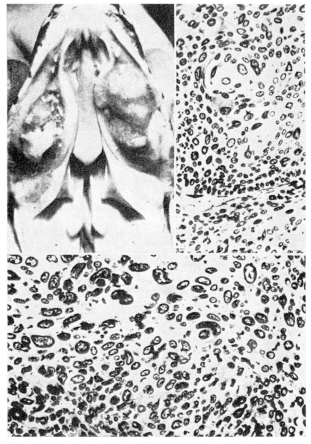

Fig. 380. Oral cancer in *Tupinambis nigropunctatus* Spix. Above left, ventral view of maxillary region; above right and below, sections through the tumour. × 211. (From Lucké and Schlumberger.)

contain bacteria of the species "*Bacterium*" *sauromali* Conti and Crawley (1939). Another tumour (Rodhain and Mettlet, 1950) contained fungal threads. It should also be mentioned that tumours may be caused through filariosis and through trematodes which encyst in reptiles. A papilloma of the gall bladder associated with a trematode infection was described by Smith and Nigrelli (1941). The same authors (1943) reported on a chelonian fibroepithelioma connected with leeches of the genus *Ozobranchus*. Smith and Coates (1938) finally found trematode eggs in the fibroepithelioma of a marine turtle.

REFERENCES

Ball, H. A. (1946). Melanosarcoma and rhabdomyoma in two pine snakes *Pituophis melanoleucus*. *Cancer Res.* 6, 134–138.

Bergmann, R. A. M. (1941). Tumoren bij Slangen. *Geneesk. Tijdschr. Ned. Ind.* 81, 547–577.

Blanchard, R. (1890). Sur une remarquable dermatose causée chez le lézard vert par un champignon du genre *Selenosporium*. *Mém. Soc. Zool., Fr.* 3, 241–255.

Bland-Sutton, J. (1885). Tumours in animals. *J. Anat. Phys.* 19, 415–475.

Conti, F. and Crawley, J. H. (1939). A new bacterial species isolated from the Chuckawalla (*Sauromalus varius*). *J. Bact.* 37, 647–653.

Kälin, J. A. (1937). Über Skeletanomalien bei Crocodiliden. *Z. Morph. Ökol. Tiere* 32, 327–437.

Klein, B. M. (1952). Die Borkengeschwulst der Eidechsen. *Mikrokosmos* 42, 49–52.

Koch, M. (1904). Demonstration einiger Geschwülste bei Tieren. *Verh. dtsch. Path. Ges.* 7, 136–147.

Lucké, B. (1938). Studies on tumours in cold-blooded vertebrates. *Ann. Rep. Tortugas Lab. Carneg. Inst. Wash.* 1937/38. 92–94.

Lucké, B. and Schlumberger, M. G. (1949). Neoplasia in cold-blooded vertebrates. *Phys. Rev.* 29, 91–216.

Nigrelli, R. F. and Smith, G. M. (1943). The occurrence of leeches, *Ozobranchus branchiatus*, in fibroepithelial tumours of marine turtles *Chelonia mydas*. *Zoologica* 2, 107–108.

Patay, R. (1933). Sur un cas d'épithélioma du rein chez *Tropidonotus natrix* (Ophidien colubridé). *C. R. Soc. Biol., Paris* 114, 65–67.

Pick, L. and Poll, M. (1903). Über einige bemerkenswerte Tumorbildungen aus der Thierpathologie, insbesondere über gutartige und krebsige Neubildungen bei Kaltblütern. *Berl. klin. Wschr.* 40, 510–572.

Plehn, M. (1911). Uber Geschwülste bei niederen Wirbeltieren. 2. *Conf.int. Étude Cancer*, 221–242.

Plimmer, M. G. (1912). Report on the deaths which occurred in the Zoological Gardens during 1911. *Proc. zool. Soc. Lond.*, 235–240.

Plimmer, M. G. (1913). Report on the deaths which occurred in the Zoological Gardens during 1912. *Proc. zool. Soc. Lond.*, 141–149.

Ratcliffe, H. L. (1935). Carcinoma of the pancreas in Say's pine snake (*Pituophis sayi*). *Amer. J. Cancer* 24, 78–79.

Ratcliffe, H. L. (1943). Neoplastic disease of the pancreas of snakes (Serpentes). *Amer. J. Path.* 19, 359–366.

Rodhain, J. and Mettlet, G. (1950). Une tumeur mycosique chez la couleuvre viperine *Tropidonotus natrix*. *Ann. Parasit.* 25, 77–79.

Schlumberger, H. G. (1953). Comparative pathology of oral neoplasms. *Oral. Surg.* 6, 1078–1094.

Schlumberger, H. G. and Lucké, B. (1948). Tumours of fishes, amphibians and reptiles. *Cancer Res.* 8, 657–754.

Schlumberger, H. G. (1958). Krankheiten der Fische, Amphibien und Reptilien. *In* "Pathologie der Laboratoriumstiere" (Cohrs, Jaffé and Meesen, eds.). Springer, Berlin, Göttingen, Heidelberg.

Schnabel, R. (1954). Papillome an einer Smaragdeidechse (*Lacerta viridis*). *Zool. Garten* **2**, 270–278.

Schwarz, F. (1923). Über zwei Geschwülste bei Kaltblütern. *Z. Krebsforsch.* **20**, 353–357.

Scott, H. H. and Beattie, J. (1927). Neoplasm in a porose crocodile. *J. Path. Bact.* **30**, 41–66.

Smith, G. M. A. and Coates, C. (1938). Fibro-epithelial growths of the skin in large marine turtles, *Chelonia mydas*. *Zoologica* **23**, 93–98.

Smith, G. M. A. (1939). The occurrence of trematode ova, *Haplotrema constrictum*, on fibroepithelial tumours of the marine turtle *Chelonia mydas*. *Zoologica* **24**, 379–389.

Smith, G. M. A. and Nigrelli, R. F. (1941). A papillomatous tumour of the gall bladder associated with infection by flukes, occurring in the marine turtle *Chelonia mydas*. *Zoologica* **26**, 13–16.

Stolk, R. (1953). Hyperkeratosis and carcinoma planocellulare in the lizard, *Lacerta agilis*. *Koninkl. Ned. Akad. Wetensch.* Ser. C. **56**, 157–163.

Stolk, R. (1958). Tumours of reptiles. Multiple osteomas in the lizard *Lacerta viridis*. *Beaufortia* **7**, 1–9.

Vaillant, B. and Pettit, A. (1902). Lesions stomacales observés chez un Python de Seba. *Bull. Mus. Hist. Nat., Paris* **8**, 593–595.

B. DISEASES DUE TO FAULTY ENVIRONMENT

Unsuitable nutrition and unsuitable environment may both cause diseases in reptiles. Animals may fall ill because they have not enough or not the right food; they may suffer from lack of sunshine, particularly from lack of u.v. radiation; or from the lack of space, and enforced immobility. Into the same group belong the harmful effects of excessive air, and soil humidity factors which frequently interfere with the health of captive reptiles.

Among the alimentary disturbances vitamin deficiencies are common but not always easily recognized. They may manifest themselves as inflammation of areas of skin or of the eyes, as oedema, difficulties in skin shedding, refusal to feed at all, oral oedema and inflammation, listlessness, fading of coloration, and an inclination to hide in the most inaccessible corner of the cage. In short, they may cause the greatest variety of symptoms and give, at first sight, no hint towards a correct diagnosis. Since small doses of vitamins are harmless and since it may take some time before the root of the trouble is discovered, it may be advisable to feed with a few drops of a multivitamin mixture wherever reptiles fail to thrive for obvious reasons. Lack of vitamin A may damage the eyes (Fig. 381), persistent softness of the carapace of tortoises is often regarded as a form of rickets due to lack of vitamin D and it must not be forgotten that, apart from the vitamin, tortoises also appreciate the addition of crushed bones to their diet. Rickets is by no means

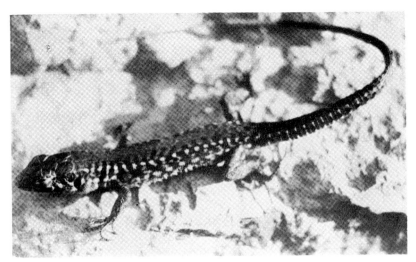

FIG. 381. *Lacerta t. taurica* Pallas imported from Greece. Oedema of eyes due to avitaminosis. Young specimen. (Photo.: Stemmler-Gyger.)

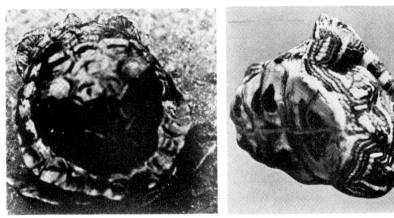

FIG. 382. Ornamental turtles affected by rickets showing distorted carapace. (Photo.: Stemmler-Morath.)

uncommon in captive animals. Hamerton and Scott, in their reports on the death of animals in a zoological garden, make repeated mention of such cases (1933 also 1926–28). Equally Kälin (1937) saw skeletal damage due to rickets in crocodiles (Fig. 382) and damage of this kind is particularly common at the end of a hibernation period when the feeding of egg-shells or crushed bone is of particular importance. Kästle (personal communication) reports that he succeeded in curing tail deformities by giving calcium and a multivitamin preparation.

Vitamin deficiency probably causes many other, not easily recognizable symptoms. Inflammatory processes of the intestinal tract (mouth and gut), so frequently seen in captive animals are, if not due to parasites, often caused by a vitamin B deficiency, and can be cured by adding this vitamin to the food.

The thyroid gland often gives cause to irregularities either in the form of hyper- or hypo-thyroidism. Hypo-thyroidism produces goitre in reptiles as well as in fish and amphibians, where, however, the condition is much more common than in reptiles. Schlumberger (1955) reported on three cases of goitre, two in tortoises and one in a lizard, all of which had been inmates of zoological gardens for several years. He suggests that the condition was caused by lack of iodine.

Since the production of vitamin D is linked up with the action of u.v. rays, environmental and metabolic factors are closely linked and interdependent. Mistakes may be aggravated by faulty or oscillating temperature or humidity.

It remains of course frequently impossible to determine the adverse environmental factors harmful to reptiles, particularly if these are found diseased in their natural environment. Fig. 383, for instance, shows an Aesculapian snake (*Elaphe l. longissima* Laur.), caught in the Tessin, with a patchy disease of the skin. No parasites were found and it was thought that the skin degeneration was caused by other noxious factors in the snake's habitat. It has to be considered, however, that the spectrum of possible parasites is a wide one and that these may not always be visible even if a hand lens is used. Animals weakened by malnutrition and/or internal parasites may eventually be killed by bacterial infection. The possible variations in the pathology of lower vertebrates are so great that we must not be surprised at the number deaths which remain undiagnosed to the last.

Into this group belong at the moment the disturbances of the equili-brium so often seen in captive *Xenopus* and the distressing *disease of the eyelids* which affects so many of the terrapins and ornamental turtles imported from overseas.

This disease was well-known to Klingelhöffer, a German ophthalmologist, who mentions, in his textbook on herpetology, that unfortunately the hard heads of terrapins were too difficult to section. And so this eye specialist who would have been so well-qualified to find the cause of this mysterious disease had to leave the work to posterity. Meanwhile he suggested that the disease was due to avitaminosis.

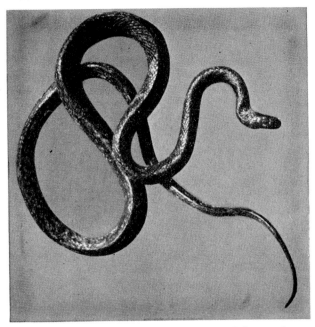

FIG. 383. *Elaphe l. longissima* from the Tessin with dermal disease, photographed soon after capture. (Photo.: Stemmler-Gyger.)

A host of different causes has, in the meantime, been blamed for this disease: faulty temperature, faulty diet, too little or too much lime in the water, bacterial infection, etc. All we know is that, while most animals die from it, some survive the disease and even regain their eyesight.

The affected specimens always belong to the genera *Clemmys*, *Emys*, *Chinemys*, *Pseudemys*, *Chrysemys* or *Pseudomedusa* and it may occur in young, freshly imported turtles or in old stock. The nictitating membrane becomes inflamed, thickened, and too easily visible with the naked eye. It closes too slowly and does not cover the eyeball quite. Its capillaries are engorged. Within a day or two first the upper, then the lower eyelid become swollen. Soon they fuse so firmly that they cannot even be separated with a blunt instrument (Fig. 384a and b). The turtle, totally blinded, mostly refuses to feed and eventually dies from inanition. But not always. Some observers have seen a hard mass eventually detaching itself from the eye, revealing a perfectly intact eyeball underneath. The disease is usually bilateral, but unilateral cases have also been seen. These animals are more likely to survive because they continue to feed.

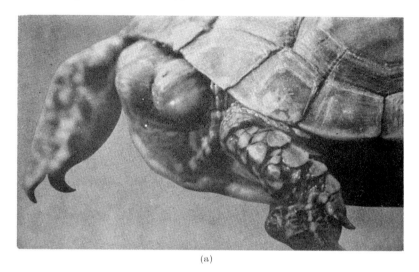

(a)

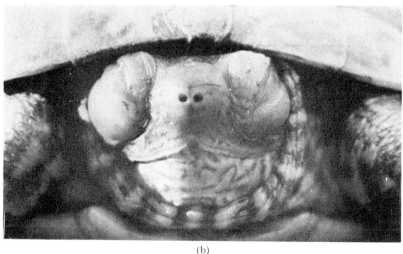

(b)

FIG. 384. *Clemmys caspica leprosa* Loveridge and Williams. Disease of the Harderian gland. (a) First week. (Photo.: E. Elkan.) (b) Anterior view.

Modern histological methods make the sectioning of turtle-heads quite feasible and the inspection of material from these cases produces a surprising result (Fig. 385). The seat of the disease is not the eyelid proper but the Harderian gland, a structure closely joined to it. The eyeball is not affected at all.

The Harderian gland, named after the Swiss anatomist Harder who discovered it in 1694 in deer, lies in the orbital cavity opposite the lachrymal gland and is present in most animals from the amphibians upwards. In man the gland is only represented by a rudimentary body, the caruncula lacrimalis. In crocodiles, snakes and the tuatara (*Sphenodon*) the lachrymal gland is missing and only the Harderian gland is developed. It has been taken for granted that it is the function of these glands to moisten and to lubricate the very vulnerable corneal surface of the eyeball. But it remained difficult to see why these glands were equally well, if not better, developed in aquatic species, whose eyes, permanently bathed in water, would not seem to need either cleaning or lubrication. The investigations of Schmidt-Nielsen and Fange (1958) have solved this enigma. These authors showed that the ophthalmic glands secrete, apart from serous fluid and a little mucus, large quantities of salt (NaCl). "Salty tears" are known well enough, but we have now learnt that, while the human kidney is quite able to excrete surplus salt without aid from any other excretory organ, the kidney of the lower vertebrate is apparently not so efficient, and we can now understand the astonishingly large size of the Harderian gland in marine animals which cannot well avoid swallowing a good deal of salt with their food.

The normal lachrymal and Harderian glands, though not identical, are of very similar structure. They are tubular acinous glands similar to the salivary glands. Statements to the effect that these glands might be sebaceous are incorrect. They are largely serous; only the excretory ducts are partly lined with goblet cells capable of producing a small amount of mucus.

Sections through the orbit of a diseased animal show the normal glandular structure completely lost. The epithelium has changed from the glandular to the squamous type; the acini are grossly dilated and distended by masses of keratinic debris which cannot be expelled (Figs. 385, 386). In short, the gland has undergone complete metaplasia, the centre being usually marked by a large accumulation of eosinophile granulocytes forming a kind of abscess. Eosinophilia is marked throughout, particularly in the liver, where capillaries and biliary ducts are surrounded by agglomerations of acidophile granulocytes. The centre of the keratinic masses in the glandular acini is usually marked by one or several degenerate nuclei, probably the remains of the original glandular epithelium.

It would be easier to explain this extraordinary histological picture
if occlusion of the excretory duct of the Harderian gland could be
demonstrated. Such an occlusion might occur in consequence of bacterial

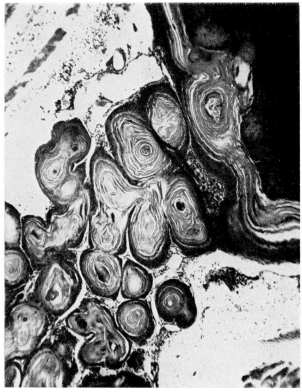

FIG. 385. *Chinemys reevesii* Gray. Section through the orbital region showing extensive
metaplasia of the Harderian gland with accumulation of keratinic masses in the acini.
Stain, Mallory. × 50. (Photo.: E. Elkan.)

infection. So far only some acid-fast mycobacteria were encountered
and these are too common and too ubiquitous to be regarded as signifi-
cant. No trace of the duct could be found in the grossly pathologic
glands and further lengthy and time-consuming research will be needed
to clarify the many problems that remain.

A signpost may be seen in the following observation. When heads of
just-hatched Malayan turtles (*Dermochelys coriacea* L.) were sectioned
the upper region of the nasal cavity was filled with numerous, so far
unidentified, nematodes. The structure of the mucous membrane was

intensely damaged by the worms. Parasites are only too often the cause of morbidity in lower vertebrates and it is by no means impossible that nematodes might obstruct the excretory ducts of the ophthalmic

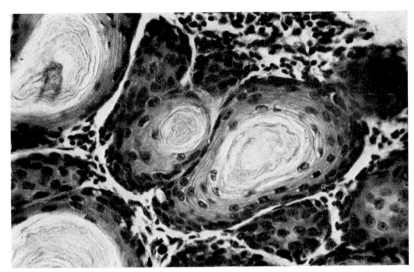

FIG. 386. As Fig. 385, × 300, showing inflammatory invasion with eosinophile granulocytes and extensive metaplasia of the Harderian gland. (Photo.: E. Elkan.)

glands. In that case the central nuclei in the keratinic masses might represent the remains of such worms. At the time of writing we can only offer this partial solution of the problem. The rest must be handed on to yet further generations of herpetologists.

Ornamental terrapins which are widely distributed as pets and rarely kept in suitable conditions often show a patchy white discoloration of the carapace accompanied by listlessness and refusal to feed. Successes obtained in treating the condition with multiple vitamin preparations make it appear very likely that the disease is caused by a form of avitaminosis. Heat, light and a variety of—preferable live—food is of the greatest importance for these small terrapins which, although sold by the thousand, are not really suitable "pets" at all.

Mertens (1927) reported on a disease of the ear and the labyrinth in a lizard (*Anolis porcatus* Gray). He noticed semispherical tumours on both sides of the head which, when opened, discharged a white chalky mass. The condition was caused by excessive chalk deposit in the saccus endolymphaticus. This sac always and quite normally contains chalk deposits in reptiles and in amphibians. The reason for the excessive deposits and the consequent distension of the sacs is not known. Krefft (1926) reported on similar "chalk tumours" and one of us (R.-K.) saw the same condition in a specimen of *Phelsuma d. dubia* Boettger (Fig. 387). Incision of the swellings again produced a thick mass which solidified on discharge.

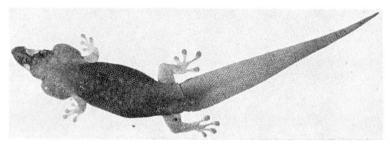

FIG. 387. *Phelsuma d. dubia* Boettger with abnormally distended chalk sacs. Eyes removed by dissection. (Orig.)

REFERENCES

Ashley, L. M. (1955). "Laboratory Anatomy of the Turtle." Wm. C. Brown publ. Dubuque. Iowa, U.S.A.

Bojanus, L. H. (1819/21). "Anatomia Testudinis Europaeae." Vilna, p. 135. Glandula lacrymalis externa. III; Illustration reprinted in Owen, R. "Anatomy of Vertebrates" (1866), Vol. I, p. 340.

Boycott, B. B. and Robins, M. W. (1961). The care of young red-eared terrapins (*Pseudemys scripta elegans*) in the laboratory. *Brit. J. Herpet.* 2, 206–210.

Franz, V. (1924). Mikroskopische Anatomie der Hilfsteile des Sehorgans der Wirbeltiere. *Erg. Anat. Entwges.* 25, 241–390.

Gegenbaur, C. (1898). "Vergleichende Anatomie der Wirbeltiere", Vol. I, Leipzig.

Graham-Jones, O. (1961). Some clinical conditions affecting the N. African tortoise ("Greek tortoise") *Testudo graeca. Vet. Rec.* 73, 371–421.

Griffiths, I. and Carter, E. (1958). Sectioning refractory animal tissue. *Stain Technology* 33, 209–214.

Hamerton, A. E. (1933). Report on deaths occurring in the Society's gardens during the year 1932. *Proc. zool. Soc. Lond.*, pp. 451–462.

Harder, J. J. (1693/4). Glandula nova lachrymalis una cum ductu secretorio in Ericiis et in Damis ab Hardere descripta. "Acta Eruditorum." publ. Lipsiae.

Harris, V. A. (1963). "The Anatomy of the Rainbow Lizard (*Agama agama* L.)." Hutchinson Trop. Monographs. London.

Hunt, T. J. (1956). Deaths of *Testudo elegans* from intestinal obstruction. *Brit. J. Herpet.* 2, 35.

Hunt, T. J. (1957). Note on diseases and mortality in testudines. *Herpetologica* 13, 19–23.

Kälin, J. A. (1937). Uber Skeletanomalieen bei Crocodiliden. *Z. Morph. Ökol. Tiere* 32, 327–347.

Kaplan, H. M. (1957). The care and diseases of laboratory turtles. *Proc. Anim. Care Panel* 7, 259–272.

Klingelhöffer, W. (1955). "Terrarienkunde", 2nd edn. Kernen, Stuttgart.

Krefft, P. (1926). "Das Terrarium", 3rd edn. Berlin.

Lever, F. V. (1954). "Histopathology of the Skin." Lippincott, Philadelphia.

Loveridge, A. (1947). Bone making material for turtles. *Copeia* 1947, p. 136.

Mertens, R. (1927). Über eine merkwürdige Erkrankung des Gehörorgans bei *Anolis* und anderen Eidechsen. *Bl. Aqu. Terrk.* **38**, 13–14.

Noble, K. (1931). "The Biology of the Amphibia." McGraw-Hill, New York.

Paule, W. J. (1953). Some comparative observations on orbital glands, with special references to the turtle. *Anat. Rec.* **115**, 408. Abstr. No. 282.

Peters, A. (1890). Beitrag zur Kenntnis der Harderschen Drüse. *Arch. mikr. Anat.* **36**.

Piersol, G. A. (1887). Beiträge zur Histologie der Harderschen Drüsen der Amphibien. *Arch. mikr. Anat.* **29**.

Pillet, A. and Bignon, F. (1885). La glande lachrymale d'une tortue géante (*Chelone viridis*). *Bull. Soc. Zool. Fr.* **10**, 60–66.

Plimmer, K. G. (1915). Reports on deaths which occurred in the Zoological Gardens during 1914 together with a list of the blood parasites found during the year. *Proc. zool. Soc. Lond.* 1915, 123–130.

Pope, C. H. (1956). "The Reptile World." Routledge and Kegan Paul, London.

Sardemann, E. (1888). Beiträge zur Anatomie der Tränendrüse. *Ber. Naturf. Ges. Freiburg* **3**, 95–128.

Schlumberger, H. G. (1955). Spontaneous goiter and cancer of the thyroid in animals. *Ohio J. Sci.* **55**, 23–43.

Schmidt-Nielsen, K. and Fange, R. (1958). Salt glands in marine reptiles. *Nature, Lond.* **182**, 781–785.

Scott, H. (1926–28). Report on the deaths occurring in the Society's gardens during the year 1925, 1926, 1927. *Proc. zool. Soc. Lond.* 1926, 231–244; 1927, 73–198; 1928, 81–119.

Schreitmüller, W. and Lederer, G. (1930). "Krankheitserscheinungen bei Fischen, Reptilien und Lurchen." Berlin.

Wallis, G. L. (1942). "The Vertebrate Eye." Cranbrook Inst. of Science, Bloomfield Hills, Michigan, U.S.A.

Weber, M. (1887). Über die Nebenorgane des Auges der Reptilien. *Arch. Nat. gesch.* **43**, 261–342.

Weichert, C. K. (1958). "The Anatomy of the Chordates." McGraw-Hill, New York.

C. Injuries through Physical Factors

Animals may suffer from excessive insolation as well as through lack of sunshine. Mosauer and Lazier (1933), examining deserticolous reptiles, found that snakes may be killed during excessively long periods of heat. Three experimental snakes were exposed to an air temperature of 35·5°C in the Coachella valley of California.

The first specimen died after 6 min with a rectal temperature of 47°C; the second after 10·5 min with a rectal temperature of 46·6°C; the third after 9 min, rectal temperature 47°C. Temperatures over 46°C were obviously fatal for these snakes. Mosauer (1936) found, furthermore, that the species *Uma notata* Baird, *Dipsosaurus dorsalis* Baird and

Girard and *Crotalus cerastes* Hallowell die once their body temperature exceeds 44·2–53°C. In the Californian deserts soil temperatures up to 62°C were observed in the morning between 9 and 15.30 h. Experimental data indicate optimal temperatures for deserticolous saurians to lie between 35 and 40°C, a rise above 45–50°C being invariably fatal. Blum and Spealman (1933) published similar findings. They found that rattlesnakes are not damaged by increased insolation as long as the temperature does not exceed the supportable limit. The snakes died as soon as the temperature of the surrounding air reached 49°C.

The reaction of reptiles to cold is similar to that of amphibians. Excessively low temperatures are particularly dangerous for aquatic specimens like turtles. Some species tolerate excessive changes badly. *Sphenodon punctatus* Gray has, according to Dawbin (1962), in its natural habitat a remarkable tolerance to varying temperatures. It still feeds at 7°C and tolerates up to 40°C in the open air.

A case of incredible tolerance to cold in terrapins has been reported by Cable (1933). He found on January 30th two specimens of *Terrapene c. carolina* L. with their heads frozen into the ice. When thawed out they seemed to be entirely undamaged. Other specimens taken from the water which had a temperature of 10°C had a body temperature as low as 9·5°C.

Reptilian species adjusted to dry and warm air do not tolerate humidity. They may also be damaged by a draughty cage or by cages the walls of which are made of particularly rough material. Cement in particular should be given a carefully smoothed surface.

REFERENCES

Blum, H. F. and Spealman, C. R. (1933). Note on the killing of rattlesnakes by "sunlight". *Copeia* **3**, 150–151.
Cable, A. R. (1933). Hibernation of the box turtle. *Copeia* **3**, 13–14.
Dawbin, W. H. (1962). The tuatara in its natural habitat. *Endeavour* **21**, Nr. 81, 16–24.
Mosauer, W. (1936). The toleration of solar heat in desert reptiles. *Ecology* **17**, 56–66.
Mosauer, W. and Lazier, E. L. (1933). Death from insolation in desert snakes. *Copeia* **3**, 149.

D. POISONING

Reptiles may be poisoned either by their keepers if chemicals are used to free cages from mites, ants or other insects, or if, in the wild, they unsuccessfully attack insects which retaliate with poisonous stings.

The modern insecticides, so popular with gardeners, are particularly harmful to small reptiles. Manufacturers (Geigy and Co. Pest Control Dept.) have issued a warning against the use of these substances for the disinfection of cages of small animals. Both snakes and lizards have proved extraordinarily sensitive to the smallest doses of DDT and many other modern insecticides under whatever alluring name they may appear. The animals die within a few hours after the slightest contact with any of these substances. The effect shows itself in loss of equilibrium, irregular muscular contractions, cramp and breathing difficulties. Very slightly poisoned specimens may recover in a water bath of several days' duration at 25–30°C, the cage temperature being raised to 30°C at the same time.

Schweizer (1952) gives exact dosage figures for insecticides where these are considered necessary to combat mites in reptile cages.

Some frogs and toads have a very effective armour in the form of poisonous skin glands. They should not be used as food for reptiles. Schreitmüller and Lederer (1930) mention fatalities caused by feeding with common toads (*B. bufo* L.).

Even where the animals have been removed from a cage and this has been cleaned and disinfected, every trace of the chemicals used should be carefully washed off before the reptiles are readmitted to their quarters. They may be sensitive to the slightest smell or a small degree of pollution of their water.

REFERENCES

Geigy and Co. Ltd. Pest Control Dept. (1947). DDT Insektizide, Reptilien und Amphibien. *Aqu. Z. Jg.* 1947, 150.
Schreitmüller, W. and Lederer, G. (1930). "Krankheitserscheinungen bei Fischen, Reptilien und Lurchen." Wenzel, Berlin.
Schweizer, H. (1952). Die Blutmilbe (*Ophionyssus natricis* Gerv. Mégn.) der "Stallfeind" des Schlangenpflegers und ihre Vernichtung. *Aqu. Terr. Z.* **5**, 103–105.

CHAPTER 22

Wound Healing and Regeneration

In the matter of wound healing and regeneration the reptiles stand somewhere midway between the Amphibia and the mammals. The topic has been dealt with by Barber (1944), Fujinami (1901) and Wallis (1927, 1938). There are also a number of accounts of fractures and their mode of healing in reptiles (Wallis, 1928; Korschelt and Stock, 1928; Korschelt, 1932; Lehmensick, 1934; Pritchard and Ruzicka, 1950).

Authors have always been interested in the regeneration of lost limbs. It was extensively discussed by Fraisse as early as 1885. The organ showing the best regenerative ability in reptiles is the tail (Korschelt, 1927/31; Slotopolsky, 1921/22). Occasionally, as shown by Werber (1905), parts of the dentigerous cranial parts may regenerate. Legs regenerate very incompletely, rarely producing more than tail-like stumps. Guyénot and Matthey (1928), Marcucci (1930) and Hellmich (1951) published a number of observations on the regeneration of the extremities in lizards. Marcucci (1930) in particular collected a great deal of material. He found that amputated toes rarely produced more than tail-like, sometimes forked stumps, sometimes no more than a short truncated appendix. Different species showed slight variations in their ability to regenerate. Regeneration in *Lacerta muralis* Laur. was found to be more complete than that in *Lacerta ocellata* Daud. Complete regeneration of a limb has never been observed in any species, nor is the regenerated part ever able to assume the function of the lost limb.

Slotopolsky (1922) studied the processes connected with the autotomy and regeneration of the lacertid tail. He showed that the vertebrae in the predestined breaking spot have a small gap which, however, does not extend to the whole cross section of the vertebra. This crack can usually be found in the sixth caudal vertebra but it may already be found in the fifth. Regeneration is subject to individual variation. The last six vertebrae are not replaced. Partial rupture and lateral incisions produce multiple regenerated buds. Dawbin (1962) pictures a forked tail in *Sphenodon punctata*.

Fractures of bones have always aroused much interest and have particularly been studied in lizards. Wallis (1927/28) maintained that the conditions of healing in reptiles varied basically from those in mammals. He worked on *Lacerta sicula* Raf. and divided the recovery period into four phases: during the first phase fibrous callus is laid down while the periosteum produces only very little of it. Hyaline

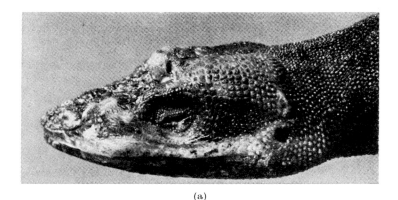

(a)

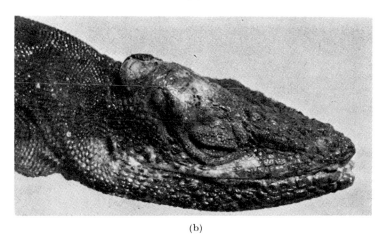

(b)

FIG. 388. *Anolis carolinensis* with a healing wound caused through biting.
(Photo.: Kästle.)

cartilaginous callus appears next, enveloping the fractured ends of the bone. The two surfaces unite by fibrous tissue. The cartilaginous callus eventually calcifies and envelops the fracture area (Fig. 388). Enchondral ossification is very slow in appearing. It goes parallel with the general calcification of the cartilaginous callus, the periostal bony callus gradually enveloping the cartilaginous parts. Fibrous callus eventually transforms itself into cartilage. Once the two fractured surfaces are united the intervening cartilage is absorbed and the cavity restored. The healing process is completely suspended if the period of hibernation intervenes and is only resumed in the following spring. Compared with events in a rat, fraçtures heal more slowly in the lizard. Cold-blooded animals produce predominantly cartilaginous callus, while bony callus is at an early stage produced in mammals. Pritchard and Ruzicka (1950) confirmed these observations and found, further, that similar conditions prevail in the frog.

REFERENCES

Barber, L. W. (1944). Correlation between wound healing and regeneration in forelimbs and tail of lizards. *Anat. Rec.* **89**, 441–451.

Dawbin, W. H. (1962). The tuatara in its natural habitat. *Endeavour* **21**, Nr. 81, 16–24.

Fraisse, B. (1885). "Die Regeneration von Geweben und Organen bei Wirbeltieren, besonders bei Amphibien und Reptilien." Kassel and Berlin.

Fujinami, A. (1901). Gewebsveränderungen bei der Heilung von Knochenfrakturen (Reptilien). *Beitr. path. Anat.* **29**, 432–485.

Guyénot, E. and Matthey, R. (1928). Les processus regénératifs dans la patte posterieure du lézard. *Roux' Arch.* **113**, 520–529.

Hellmich, G. (1951). A case of limb regeneration in the Chilean iguanid *Liolaemus*. *Copeia* 1951, 241–242.

Korschelt, E. (1927/31). "Regeneration und Transplantation." Berlin.

Korschelt, E. (1932). Über Frakturen und Skeletanomalieen der Wirbeltiere. II. Vögel, Reptilien, Amphibien und Fische. *Beitr. path. Anat.* **89**, 668–717.

Korschelt, E. and Stock, H. (1928). "Geheilte Knochenbrüche bei wildlebenden und in Gefangenschaft gehaltenen Tieren." Berlin.

Lehmensick, R. (1934). Über Panzerverletzungen bei Schildkröten. *Zool. Anz.* **105**, 325–331.

Marcucci, E. (1930). Il potere rigenerativo degli arti nei rettili. *Arch. zool. Ital.* **14**, 227–252.

Pritchard, J. J. and Ruzicka, A. J. (1950). Comparison of fracture repair in the frog, lizard and rat. *J. Anat.* **84**, 236–261.

Slotopolsky, B. (1921/22). Beiträge zur Kenntnis der Verstümmelungs- und Regenerationsvorgänge am Lacertilierschwanz. *Zool. Jahrb. Anat.* **43**, 219–322.

Wallis, K. (1927). Zur Knochenhistologie und Kallusbildung beim Reptil (*Clemmys leprosa*). *Z. Zellforsch.* **6**, 1–26.

Wallis, K. (1928). Über den Knochenkallus beim Kaltblüter (Eidechse). *Z. Zellforsch.* **7**, 257–289.

Werber, J. (1905). Regeneration der Kiefer bei der Eidechse *Lacerta agilis*. *Roux' Arch.* **19**, 248–258.

CHAPTER 23

Developmental Abnormalities

Under this heading we shall have to consider the appearances of double and multiple monsters as well as abnormal development of single organs, albinism and melanism.

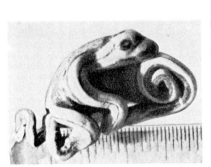
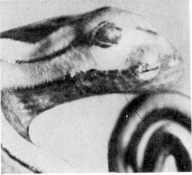

FIG. 389. Siamese twins in *Anguis fragilis* L. Head and body joined down to the last third of the body. (Photo.: Stemmler-Gyger.)

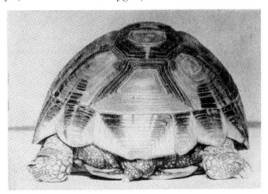

FIG. 390. Anomaly in the development of the carapace of a Greek tortoise *Testudo h. hermanni* Gmelin with unpaired supracaudal scale (typical of *T. graeca* L.) and incised edge of carapace (typical of *T. marginata* Schoepff). (From Wermuth.)

Double monsters have frequently been seen in chelonians. Hilde-brand (1930, 1938) described cases with double heads, double tails as well as complete or incomplete "Siamese twins". Into the former category belonged a pair of *Pseudemys floridana* Le Conte, the twins being united by the posterior part of the ventral shield only. Another pair, in this case of *"Chrysemys scaber"*, were joined laterally.

Fig. 389 shows the remarkable case of a slow-worm (*Anguis fragilis* L.) brought to our notice by the kindness of O. Stemmler of Basle. Here we have two complete animals endowed with only one head. The opposite malformation, where one body carries two heads, seems to be more common in snakes. Willis (1932) reported on a double embryo in a lizard.

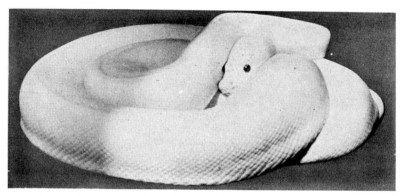

FIG. 391. *Python molurus* from India. Albinotic specimen with black-blue eyes. Specimen in the collection of the Mus. Nat. Hist. Bern. (Photo.: Stemmler-Gyger.)

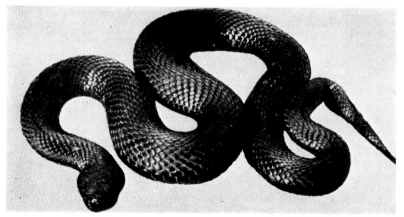

FIG. 392. *Vipera aspis aspis* L. caught at Innertkirchen Switzerland. Melanotic female. (Photo.: Stemmler-Gyger.)

Among other deformations may be seen truncation of the head, malformation of the mouth and deficiencies in the dentigerous bones. Kälin (1937) saw such cases in crocodiles, all caused by skeletal anomalies. Wermuth (1961) described an anomaly in a specimen of *Testudo h. hermanni* Gmelin, the Greek tortoise. The animal had a single supra-caudal scale which is typical for *T. graeca* L. and a serrated edge of the carapace which is typical for *T. marginata* Schoepff (Fig. 390). Anomalies of the carapace are fairly common in chelonians (Mertens, 1936). They may be combined with other abnormal developments.

Albinotic animals are most striking among colour deviations in reptiles (Fig. 391). Melanism, the opposite, also occurs frequently (Fig. 392). Schetty (1950) reported on a melanotic lizard (*Lacerta viridis viridis* Laur.).

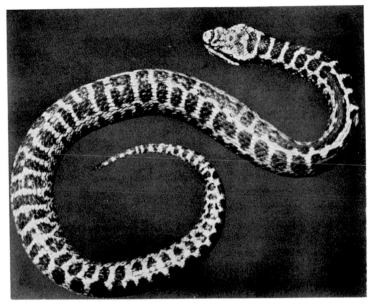

Fig. 393. One-year-old specimen of *Vipera aspis aspis* L. with two separate dorsal rows of patches. (Photo.: Bertolf.)

It seems doubtful whether the appearance of accessory parietal organs described for instance by Haffner (1955) for *Lacerta vivipara* Jaquin should be included among the anomalies since they are extraordinarily common in reptiles, particularly so in lizards. Haffner himself found such rudimentary eyes in one-sixth of his material. Attempts at lens and retina formation can clearly be seen in these organs which, in some

cases, are paired and often connected with the mesencephalon by a
thin strand of optic nerve. There is always a gap in the bony skull

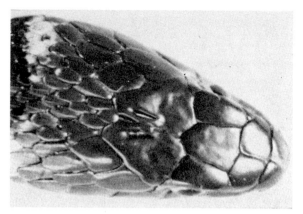

Fig. 394. Dorsal view of the head of a *Natrix natrix* L. with one central and two
lateral parietal fossae. (Photo.: E. Elkan.)

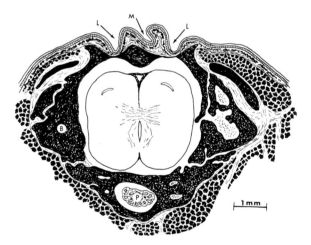

Fig. 395. Transverse section through the skull of the grass snake shown in Fig. 394.
Note the extreme attenuation of the bony brain capsule opposite the two lateral grooves
(*L*). There is no corresponding attenuation opposite the median groove (*M*). *B*, brain
capsule; *P*, pituitary gland. Drawn by microprojection. (E. Elkan.)

dorsal to the parietal eye, matched in some cases by a pitted scale or a
pair of pitted scales on the surface. As shown in Fig. 394 these gaps
can appear in a variety of patterns. The grass snake in question—
probably a great rarity—had two parietal and one median groove.

When, during a period of hibernation, the snake died, sections were made through the head. These showed extreme attenuation of the bone opposite the trough of the lateral dermal grooves. At the level of the median groove the bone was unaffected. No abnormality of the brain could be seen and we are left to speculate on the phylogenetic significance of this syndrome (Fig. 395).

Hermaphroditic sexual organs are of more obvious teratological interest. Risley (1941) reported on a specimen of *Chrysemys picta marginata* Agassiz which proved to be a complete hermaphrodite equipped with two testicles, a well-developed left oviduct and nine oocytes in the right and thirty-two in the left testis. Another turtle (*Malaclemys terrapin centrata* Latreille) showed some degree of female pseudohermaphroditism. The juvenile animal was equipped with ovaries and an ovarian medullary tumour composed of testicular tissue.

We owe further observations on chelonian hermaphrodites to Fantham (1905) and Matthey (1927). Fantham reported on a Greek tortoise (*T. graeca* L.) which developed a complete male genital system and mature oocytes. Matthey's specimen (*Emys orbicularis* L.) had hermaphroditic gonads, an oviduct and parts of the male copulatory organ.

Lantz (1923) saw a hermaphroditic specimen of *Lacerta saxicola defilippi* Cam. Judging by the number of cases reported, hermaphroditism is rarer in reptiles than in amphibians and fish.

Forbes (1941) tried to influence the sex of reptiles artificially. He inserted peritoneal implants of cristalline testosterone or oestroform into specimens of *Sceloporus spinosus floridanus* Stejn. After 6½ weeks the animals showed testicular atrophy, hyperplasia of the Müllerian ducts and hypertrophy of the epididymis and the vasa deferentia. Oestroform implantation produced testicular atrophy with loss of spermatogenesis, atrophy of spermatic ducts and the epididymis and hyperplasia of the Müllerian ducts.

REFERENCES

Clay, W. M. (1935). The occurrence of albinos in a brood of the common water snake *Natrix sipedon. Copeia* 1935, 115.

Cunningham, B. (1937). "Axial Bifurcation in Serpents." Durham.

Dawbin, W. H. (1962). The tuatara in its natural habitat. *Endeavour* **21**, No. 81, 16–24.

Fantham, H. B. (1905). On hermaphroditism and vestigial structures in the reproductive organs of *Testudo graeca. Amer. Mag. Nat. Hist.* 7 ser. **16**, 120–125.

Forbes, T. R. (1941). Observations on the urogenital anatomy of the adult male lizard *Sceloporus* and on the action of implanted pellets of testosterone and of oestrone. *J. Morph.* **68**, 71–69.

Glaesner, L. (1924). Über drei Doppelbildungen von *Chelonia mydas. Zool. Anz.* **60**, 185–194.

Haffner, K. v. (1955). Über accescorische Parietalorgane und Nebenparietalaugen als degenerative Bildungen am Parietalauge. *Mitt. Hamb. Zool. Mus. Inst.* **53**, 25–32.

Hildebrandt, S. F. (1930). Duplicity and other abnormalities in diamond-back terrapins. *J. Elisha Mitchell Sci. Soc.* **46**, 41–53.

Kälin, J. A. (1937). Über Skeletanomalien bei Crocodiliden. *Z. Morph. Ökol. Tiere* **32**, 327–347.

Lantz, L. A. (1923). Hermaphroditisme partiel chez *Lacerta saxicola. Bull. Soc. Zool. Fr.* **48**, 289–290.

Matthey, R. (1927). Intersexualité chez une tortue (*Emys europea*). *C.R. Soc. Biol., Paris* **97**, 369–371.

Mertens, R. (1936). Eine bemerkenswerte Variation des Schildkrötenpanzers. "*Isis*" *Mitt. München Jg.* 1934/36, 15–19.

Meisenheimer, J. (1930). "Geschlecht und Geschlechter im Tierreich". Vol. II, Fischer, Jena.

Müller, L. (1927). Neigung zum Melanismus bei Reptilien von der Insel Milos. *Bl. Aqu. Terrk.* **38**, 217–273.

Procter, J. B. (1926). A note on an albino Grass-snake. *Proc. zool. Soc. Lond.*, 1095–1096.

Risley, P. L. (1950). Some observations on hermaphroditism in turtles. *J. Morph.* **68**, 101–119.

Schetty, P. (1950). Eine melanotische Smaragdeidechse *Lacerta v. viridis* Laur. *Wschr. Aqu. Terrk.* **44**, 278–280.

Schweizer, H. (1951). Über eine der *Vipera aspis hugyi* Sehinz sehr nahestehende südalpine Population von *Vipera aspis aspis* L. *Aqu. Terr. Z.* **4**, 78–81.

Wermuth H. (1961). Anomalien bei einer griechischen Landschildkröte (*Testudo hermanni hermanni* Gmelin). *S.B. Ges. naturf. Fr. Berl.* N.F. **1**, 139–142.

Willis, R. A. (1932). A monstrous twin embryo in a lizard, *Tiliqua scincoides. J. Anat.* **66**, 189–201.

CHAPTER 24

The Organic Systems of Reptiles and their Importance in Reptilian Pathology

This chapter makes an attempt to classify the diseases of reptiles according to the organs in which they occur, particularly with a view to the fact that disease of one organ can have the most varied effects on others and on the animal as a whole.

We are helped in this task by the reports issued by those in charge of large animal collections like the London Zoo, which issues annual reports on the deaths of the animals in the Gardens and their causes.

Since our table can hardly hope to be complete even at the time of writing and since the science of animal pathology is undergoing a period of rapid growth, the reader who is interested in detail will want to refer to the wealth of original papers published in the journals of pathology and zoology of all countries.

The surface may be affected by injuries, swelling, tumours, inflammations, infestation by worms and mites or by avitaminosis. Discoloration may be congenital or, particularly in the case of inflammation, a sign of serious illness.

The intestinal canal is, of all the organic systems, the one most exposed to disease. Hunt (1957), investigating the cause of death in chelonians, found diseases of the gut to be responsible in 40% of his cases. Of these again most concerned the stomach and the intestine which were frequently infected by amoebae, sometimes by faulty feeding, occasionally by avitaminosis. Faulty nourishment combined with lack of exercise tends to produce constipation in captive animals. Hunt mentions (1956) the case of a *Pseudemys scripta elegans* Wied. which died from intestinal obstruction after having eaten the seed of *Curica papaya* L. The large intestine was stretched to capacity and on the point of rupturing.

The respiratory organs are almost equally exposed to disease. In Hunt's (1957) statistic they supplied 35% of all deaths in chelonians, including inflammation, abscesses and gangrene. Pulmonary atelectasis, a state in which the lungs are collapsed and contain no air, was described by Schreitmüller and Lederer (1930). Just as in amphibians, mycoses, aspergilloses and infection with acid-fast cold-water bacilli play their part and are very likely to gain entry through the bronchi or the lungs.

The blood, if diseased, will probably be found to be invaded by Protozoa, filaria, trematodes or other parasites.

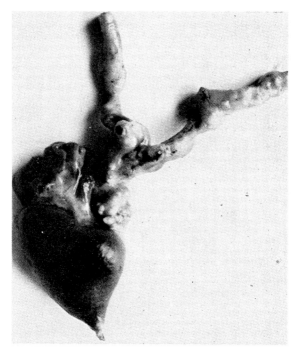

Fig. 396. *Iguana iguana* L. Heart and main blood vessels with extensive deposits of cholesterol. (Photo.: W. Frank.)

The skeletal system is much exposed to disease and deformation.

Osteomalacia and osteoporosis may appear in consequence of lack of vitamin D and of enteritis (Wallis, 1927). Osteogenetic tumours have also been described.

The urogenital system, though not as exposed as the other organs, may be the seat of disease. Hunt (1927) mentions cases of fatal nephritis in turtles. Nephrolithiasis is more commonly seen in tortoises. In very dry surroundings these sometimes fail to void their urine, a condition which may lead to autointoxication. Cases of excessive deposition of urates resembling gout have been seen by Appleby and Giller (1960). They reported on nine cases of urate deposits in joints, the liver and the heart (cf. Zwart, 1963, and Fig. 397). We owe to the kindness of Dr. W. Frank, Stuttgart, the picture (Fig. 396) of a large lizard (*Iguana iguana*) with excessive deposits of cholesterol in the walls of the large blood vessels. The same author provided the picture of the heart of a gavial which suffered from severe gout. This animal died when the heart was entirely encrusted with deposits of uric acid (Fig. 397).

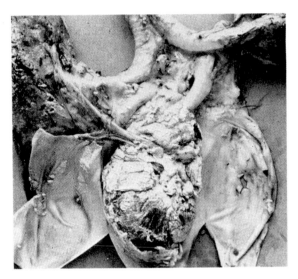

Fig. 397. Malay gavial (*Tomistoma schlegali*) suffering from severe gout. Heart and main blood vessels encrusted with uric acid deposits. (Photo.: W. Frank.)

Diseases of the sexual system concern particularly the eggs (Hunt's (1957) egg-necrosis) or the ovary. Klingelhöffer (1955) mentions the dangerous situation which arises when the process of oviposition is disturbed. This condition affects many captive reptilians, particularly tortoises and chameleons, and is probably due to a combination of causes. At the time of writing any attempt at treatment seems to be as dangerous as the condition itself.

Of the sensory organs the eye disease of terrapins is by far the most commonly seen. Since there have been no reports on this disease in wild animals it must be due to factors connected with captivity. Infection of the excretory ducts of the Harderian gland is the most likely cause, but it remains difficult to explain why in one and the same cage some of the specimens should contract the disease and others not.

REFERENCES

Appleby, E. C. and Giller, W. G. (1960). Some cases of gout in reptiles. *J. Path. Bact.* **30**, 427–430.

Hamerton, A. E. (1935). Report on deaths occurring in the Society's gardens during the year 1932. *Proc. zool. Soc. Lond.* 1935, 451–482.

Hunt, T. J. (1956). Deaths of *Testudo elegans* from intestinal obstruction. *Brit. J. Herpet.* **2**, 35.

Hunt, T. J. (1957). Notes on diseases and mortality in testudines. *Herpetologica* **13**, 19–23.

Klingelhöffer, W. (1959). "Terrarienkunde." 2nd edn. Kernen, Stuttgart.

Schreitmueller, W. and Lederer, G. (1930). "Krankheitserscheinungen bei Fischen, Reptilien und Lurchen." Wenzel, Berlin.

Scott, H. (1926–28). Report on the deaths occurring in the Society's gardens during the years 1925, 1926, 1927. *Proc. zool. Soc. Lond.* 1926, 231–244; 1927, 173–198; 1928, 81–119.

Wallis, K. (1927). Zur Knochenhistologie und Kallusbildung beim Reptil (*Clemys leprosa* Schweigg.). *Z. Zellforsch.* **6**, 1–16.

Zwart, P. (1963). Studies on Renal Pathology in Reptiles. Diss. Utrecht.

CHAPTER 25

Table of Localization, Symptoms and Possible Causes of Diseases in Reptiles

Localization	Symptoms	Possible causes
Skin and carapace	Small tumours	Cold-water tuberculosis, fungi
	Abscesses	Filariae; dracunculids
	Larger tumours	Filariae; malignancy
	Hyperkeratosis	Mites; fungi
	Oedema; ulceration	Mites; blood filariae
	Softening of carapace	Avitaminosis; faulty feeding
Eye	Blindness	Disease of the Harderian gland; infection
Mouth	Mouth permanently open	Inflammation of mucous membrane; blockage of nasal passage; nematodes; lack of vitamins
	Mouth containing cheesy masses	Intestinal disease
Intestines	Inflammation	Flagellates; sporozoa; ciliates; entamoeba; helminths; avitaminosis; faulty nutrition
	Prolapse	Constipation
Extremities	Solid tumours; difficulties in movements	Gout
Liver and gall bladder	White foci	Sporozoa; tuberculosis; malignancy; fungus infection
Peritoneal cavity	Ascites, clear or sanguinous	Any severe systemic disease and infection; congestion of liver; ovarian necrosis; helminthiasis
Skeleton	Softening or brittleness of bones; malformation; bony tumours	Faulty feeding; avitaminosis D; Malignant disease
Lungs; trachea; bronchi	Inflammation; obstruction; atelectasis	Bacterial infection; parasitic worms

Localization	Symptoms	Possible causes
Circulatory system and heart	Circulating blood parasites	Filaria;dracunculids;trematodes
	Obstruction of blood vessels	Trypanosoma
	Intracellular parasites	Haemosporidia; Adeleidea; Piroplasma
Muscles and nerves	Tumours	Parasitic protozoa
Sexual organs	Degeneration; atrophy	Sporozoa; obstructed oviposition
Kidney	Degeneration; urate deposits	Faulty metabolism; parasitic fungi and Protozoa
Urinary bladder	Inflammation	Trematodes
General symptoms	Listlessness; apathy	Metabolic disturbances; parasites; faulty temperature or humidity; lack of sunshine; unsuitable cage
	Growth disturbances	Irregularities of the endocrine system

CHAPTER 26

Treatment

A. DRUGS*

Drug	Application	Diagnosis
Alcohol, diluted	External, with brush	White spots in turtles
Antibiotics	Mixed with food	Infections
Borax solution	External as drops	Eye infections
Chinosol	Solution, as bath	Inflammation of mouth
Chloramphenicol	Oral or added to the water	*Aeromonas hydrophila*
Chlorcamphor sol.	External	Mites
Cuprex	Solution	Disinfection of cages
Enterovioform	Mixed with food	Amoebiasis
Formalin	5–10% solution	Disinfection of cages; preservation of dead specimens
Gammexan	External, with brush	Mites
Helminal	Mixed with food	Helminths
Iodine	External, with brush	Skin injuries
Cod liver oil, also as ointment	External	Parasites
	Internal	Rickets
Lugol's solution	External, with brush	Skin defects and inflammation
Nematolyt-Vet.	With food	Helminthiasis
Paraffin liqu.	1 ml per anum	Constipation
Protargol	5% sol. as eye drops or bath	Ophthalmic inflammations
Castor oil	1 : 1 with absol. alcohol, external, with brush	Mites
Salt (NaCl)	Mild solutions as bath	White spots in turtles
Santonin	Very small doses with food every 6–7 days	Helminthiasis
Socatyl (Ciba)	Solution in water	Diarrhoea
Sulphanilamide	Solution: externally	Inflammation of the eyes Inflammation of the mouth
Proflavin emulsion	Externally	Skin defects and inflammation
Vitamin drugs f.i. Vigartol	Mix with food	Avitaminosis

* The table can only give some preliminary hints at the use of drugs. Treatment by physical means is discussed under section B.

B. Biological and Physical Methods of Treatment

Wherever possible these methods should be preferred to treatment with drugs or chemicals. They include strict imitation of natural surroundings including soil, opportunities for climbing and hiding, provision of clean water of suitable temperature, control of general air temperature and humidity, air currents and nutrition. It can be seen from this list that the task of producing ideal conditions for captive reptiles is by no means an easy one. Where it is fulfilled however the keeper may well claim that the animals in his care are better provided for than they ever would be in their natural surroundings which may well be lacking in one or several of the conditions mentioned. It is also obvious that, just as we cannot keep tropical and arctic plants in the same hothouse, reptiles from different habitats cannot be accommodated in one and the same cage. Nor should it be taken for granted that several members of the same species will live in eternal peace with each other. They may do so for a while and deceive the keeper until he is one morning faced with the results of a great fight, the reasons for which he will never learn.

There is an extensive literature on the choice and preparation of suitable foods for captive reptiles. Some species will adapt themselves to substitutes where the natural food cannot be supplied. Others are entirely unadaptable and no attempt should be made to keep them in cages where they will only succumb to a lingering death from starvation. It is perhaps not surprising to notice that the larger a reptile at the time of its capture the more depressing is the effect of captivity on its appetite. Snakes so afflicted may starve for months and may then suddenly, and for no obvious reasons, break their fast and develop a perfectly normal appetite. The fact that they can usually be seen lying coiled up under or over the source of heat shows the importance of such installations, nor should the provision of water baths be neglected in purely terrestrial animals. An occasional water spray, depositing dew drops on plants, is a useful adjunct. Like the Amphibia the reptiles have an enormous tenacity of life and there must be many specimens in collections which have outlived generations of their keepers.

Chapter 27

Reptilia and Human Hygiene

In a few cases it is just possible that reptiles may transmit diseases to man. This applies particularly to *Salmonella* infections, where it is however rarely possible to assert with certainty in which direction the infection was transmitted, since both humans and reptiles may carry the infection without showing signs of disease. Children playing with captive pets are of course most likely to infect themselves in this way, and there have been several reports of outbreaks of salmonellosis in homes with freshly imported turtles or tortoises.

Bartonella bacilliformis Strong, which causes Oroya fever in S. America, is suspected of being carried by reptiles, from whom it is transferred to humans by *Phlebotomus* flies.

Ticks, particularly the genera *Amblyomma* and *Ornithodoros*, undoubtedly play a part in transmitting diseases in the countries where they occur. *O. talaje* Guérin-Menéville, for instance, transmits the American relapsing fever, *Amblyomma* species *Rickettsiae*. The Tsutsugamushi disease and the scrub typhus are equally transmitted by mites, particularly a *Trombicula* species, which sucks blood from lizards and humans.

The question of the transmissibility of virus diseases by reptiles has lately been studied in America. Thomas and Ecklund (1962) succeeded in transmitting the WEE (Western Equine Encephalomyelitis) virus to snakes with the aid of the mosquito *Culex tarsalis*. The virus remained viable in the snakes (*Thamnophis ordinoides* Baird and Girard) for some time. The importance of this procedure lies in the fact that the disease does not only affect horses but may be transferred to humans.

The trypanosomes and malarial parasites infesting reptiles are species specific and, vice versa, reptiles do not admit human blood parasites.

Of helminths (nematodes) only *Gnathostoma* species might be transmitted from reptiles to humans. *Gnathostoma spinigerum* Owen, which occurs in S.E. Asia, produces oedema of the skin, particularly in the face and the hands. The first intermediate hosts are *Cyclops* spp., the second fish, frogs and aquatic snakes of undetermined species. The remaining reptilian helminths do not seem transmissible to man.

The rightly feared common blood mite of snakes (*Ophionyssus natricis*) may occasionally be transferred to humans. Cases have been reported of workers dealing with infested snakes suffering from itching skin lesions. The common tick of sheep may infest other mammals and man and has also been found on some of the larger tropical species of snakes.

The tick *Hyalomma* (now *Hyalommasta*) *aegyptium* L. 1758 is not indigenous to northern countries but is frequently imported attached to tortoises which are unfortunately still regularly imported as pets in great numbers. The tick, according to Arthur (1963), has not so far established itself in England but biologists have been suspicious of its supposed ability to migrate to mammals like hedgehogs, donkeys, hamsters and dogs. It has also been suspected of transmitting bovine piroplasmosis and other diseases but further verification of these observations is required. So far as the buyers of tortoises are concerned they are well advised to inspect new purchases thoroughly for the presence of ticks. They can easily be dealt with by a little D.D.T. powder or a drop of methylated spirit. It is not advisable to try to remove the live tick from the tortoise; once killed it will shrivel up and fall off spontaneously.

REFERENCES

Arthur, D. R. (1963). "British Ticks." Butterworths, London.
Thomas, L. A. and Eklund, C. M. (1962). Overwintering of Western Equine Encephalomyelitis virus in Garter snakes experimentally infected by *Culex tarsalis*. *Proc. Soc. exp. Biol.*, *N.Y.* **109**, 421–424.

notes

GLOSSARY I

Zoological Names, Trivial Names and Main Habitat of Species Mentioned in the Text

Most names in the glossary are taken from the "List of the Vertebrated Animals",
Vol. III, published by the Zoological Society of London in 1929.

Zoological names	Trivial names	Main habitat
Acanthodactylus erythrurus (= *A. vulgaris*)	Spanish fringe-fingered lizard	Southwest Europe, North Africa
Abramis brama	Bream	Fresh waters of North and Central Europe
Acerina cernua	Ruffe or Pope	Fresh waters of Europe
Acipenser sturio	Sturgeon	European seas. Atlantic coast of N. America
Agama adramitana		North Africa
Agama stellio	Hardoun. Starred lizard	Middle East, Asia Minor, Egypt
Agkistrodon piscivorus	Cotton-mouth moccassin Water moccassin	West Virginia, Florida, Gulf States, Southern N. America
Alburnus alburnus	Bleak	Fresh waters of North and Central Europe
Alytes obstetricans	Midwife toad	Southern Europe. Spain
Ambystoma tigrinum	Tiger salamander Larval form: Axolotl	Southern U.S.A., Mexico
Ameiurus nebulosus	Dwarf catfish	Fresh waters of North America
Ameiva ameiva	Surinam lizard	South and Central America
Amia calva	Bowfin	Lakes and swamps of North America
Amphisbaena alba	White burrowing lizard Red worm lizard	Brazil
Amphiuma	Blind eel (amphibian)	Southern States of the U.S.A.
Amyda (= *Trionyx*) *ferox*	Fierce soft-shelled turtle	S.E. U.S.A., S. Carolina to Florida and Louisiana
Amyda (= *Trionyx*) *spinifera*	Spiny soft-shelled turtle	Southern States of North America
Anabantidae	Labyrinth fishes	Fresh waters of Southern Asia and Africa
Anarrhichas lupus	Sea wolf	Seas of Northern Europe and America
Anguilla anguilla	Eel	Rivers of Europe. Atlantic ocean
Anguis fragilis	Slow-worm	Europe, Western Asia, North-West Africa, Eastern Siberia
Anolis equestris	Greater Cuban anolis lizard	West Indies, Cuba

Zoological names	Trivial names	Main habitat
Anolis porcatus	A lizard	South-Eastern States of U.S.A., Cuba
Anoptichthys jordani	Blind characid fish	Mexican caves
Aphanius	Top minnow	Spain, Italy, Near East
Aplodinotus grunniens	American freshwater drum	Guatemala to Canada
Argulus foliaceus	Fish louse	Parasitic on fish
Asellus aquaticus	Water louse. Sow bug	Fresh waters, Europe
Aspis cerastes	Horned viper	North Africa
Barbus barbus	Barbel	Fresh waters, Europe
Basiliscus vittatus	Banded basilisk (Lizard)	Central America
Betta splendens	Regan's Siamese fighting fish	Fresh waters of Siam and the Malay States
Bitis arietans (= *Bitis lachesis*)	Puff adder	Africa, from Morocco to Cape of Good Hope
Bitis nasicornis	Nose-horned viper	West Africa, Liberia, Gabon, Congo
Blicca björkna	White bream	Fresh waters, Temperate zone
Boaedon f. fuliginosus	Sooty snake	Africa
Boaedon lineatus	African lined snake	Africa
Bombina	Fire-bellied toad	Europe
Bothrops jararaca (= *Bothrops atrox*)	Fer-de-lance (snake)	Central and South America, Trinidad, Martinique, St. Lucia, Tobago
Bufo americanus	Northern toad	Eastern North America
Bufo bufo (= *B. vulgaris*)	Common toad	Europe, Temperate Asia
Bufo boreas	Mountain toad. Californian toad	Western North America
Bufo calamita	Natterjack	Europe
Bufo lentiginosus (= *B. americanus*)	American toad	Eastern North America
Bufo marinus	Giant toad. Marine toad	Tropical America
Bufo melanostictus	Indian toad, Common Asiatic toad	India, Tropical Asia, Malay States
Bufo regularis	Common African toad	Africa
Bufo valliceps	Helmet-headed toad	Southern part of U.S.A., Mexico
Bufo viridis	Green toad	Europe, North Africa, Western Asia
Bulimus	A water snail	Europe
Callorhynchus	Plow-nosed or Elephant-chimaera	Southern oceans, New Zealand, Tasmania
Carassius carassius	Goldfish. Crucian carp	Fresh waters of Europe and N.E. Asia
Cardium edule	Common cockle	European marine waters
Caretta caretta	Loggerhead turtle	Tropical and subtropical seas
Carnegiella strigata	Hatchet belly	South America, Panama to La Plata
Causus lichtensteini	West African viper	West Africa

Zoological names	Trivial names	Main habitat
Causus rhombeatus	Night adder. Cape viper	Tropical and South Africa
Centrarchidae	Sunfishes	Eastern North America
Ceramodactylus doriae	A lizard	Persia, Arabia
Chalcides ocellatus	Eyed skink	Morocco, Egypt, S.W. Asia, S. Europe
Chelodina longicollis	Long-necked terrapin Snake tortoise	South and S.E. Australia
Chelonia mydas (= *Ch. viridis*)	Green turtle	Tropical and subtropical seas, Ascension island
Chelydra serpentina	Snapping turtle, Alligator terrapin	Eastern North America
Chimaera monstrosa	Rabbit fish	Temperate zone of Atlantic ocean
Chinemys reevesii	Chinese turtle	China, Japan. Fresh waters and swamps
Chitra indica	Long-headed soft-shelled turtle	Northern India, Burma, Siam, Malay peninsula
Chrysemys picta	Painted terrapin	Eastern North America
Chrysolophus amhersti	Lady Amherst's pheasant	Szechuan, West China, East Tibet
Clarias	Amphibious catfish	Fresh and brackish waters of S.E. Asia
Clemmys caspica leprosa	Caspian terrapin	Western Asia, S.E. Europe, Persia, Mesopotamia, Cyprus, Crete
Clemmys guttata	Speckled terrapin	Eastern North America
Clemmys japonica	Japanese terrapin, Ishigame	Japan
Clemmys leprosa	Spanish terrapin	Iberian peninsula, N.W. Africa, Senegambia
Clupea harengus	Herring	North Atlantic and North Pacific Ocean, Channel, Baltic sea
Cnemidophorus lemniscatus	Strand race runner	Tropical America
Colisa lalia	Dwarf gourami (a fish)	Fresh waters of Northern India
Coluber constrictor	Racer. American black snake	North America
Coluber flagellum	Coach whip snake	North America
Coluber gemonensis (= *Coluber jugularis*)	European whip snake	Southern Europe, S.W. Asia, Western Persia
Coluber radiatus (= *Elaphe radiata*)	Rayed snake	India, S.W. Asia, Southern China, Malay States
Conger conger	Conger eel	Marine, world-wide
Conolophus subcristatus	Galapagos land iguana	Galapagos and Seymour Islands
Constrictor constrictor	Boa constrictor	South America, Brazil, Venezuela, N.E. Peru, Guianas
Cordylus (= *Zonurus*) *giganteus*	Girdled lizard	South Africa

Zoological names	Trivial names	Main habitat
Coregonus vandesius	Whitefish	Great lakes of North America
Corydoras paleatus	Coat-of-mail catfish	Fresh waters, Eastern South America
Crenicichla	Pike cichlids	Fresh waters, Eastern South America
Crocodilus niloticus	Nile crocodile	North-East Africa, Madagascar
Crocodilus palustris	Marsh crocodile	India, Burma, Baluchistan
Crocodilus porosus	Estuarine crocodile	East India, Ceylon, South China, N. Australia, Solomon and Fiji islands
Crotalus cerastes	Horned rattlesnake, Sidewinder	Western North America, California, Arizona
Crotaphopeltis (= *Leptodeira*) *hotamboiea*	Rufescent snake	Southern and tropical Africa
Crypturus noctivagus	Banded Tinamon Bird	Eastern Brazil
Ctenosaurus acanthura	Spring-tailed iguana	Southern States of N. America, Mèxico
Cyclanorbis senegalensis	Senegal soft-shelled turtle	Tropical Africa
Cynops pyrrhogaster	Japanese newt	Japan
Cyprinus carpio	Carp	Fresh waters, Europe, Temperate Asia
Cystobranchus mammillatus	Burbot leech	Fresh waters, Temperate zones
Cystobranchus respirans	Barbel leech	Fresh waters, Temperate zones
Dasypeltis scaber	Egg eating snake, Rough-keeled snake	Africa. Cape province to Egypt and Abyssinia
Dendraspis angusticeps	Green mamba	South and tropical Africa, Kenya, Angola
Dendrophis calligaster solomonensis	A snake	Solomon islands
Dermochelys coriacea	Giant leatherback turtle	Tropical seas, Malaya
Desmognathus fuscus	Northern dusky salamander	North America
Diemyctilus viridescens	Red-spotted newt	North America
Diploglossus	Galliwasp lizard	Central America
Dipsadoboa unicolor	Gunther's green snake	West Africa, Sierra Leone, Congo
Dipsadomorphus irregularis	A snake	Celebes, Moluccas, Papuasia, Solomon Islands
Dipsosaurus dorsalis	Desert pygmi iguana	California
Discoglossus pictus	Painted frog	South Europe, Spain, N.W. Africa
Draco volans	Flying lizard	Indo-China, Burma, Malay States, Philippines
Dromophis lineatus	A snake	Tropical Africa
Drymarchon corais	Gopher or Corais snake	Southern U.S.A., Brazil, Bolivia

Zoological names	Trivial names	Main habitat
Echis carinata	Carpet viper	N. Africa, S.W. Asia, India, Ceylon, Egypt
Elaphe flavolineata	Common Malayan racer	Malay States
Elaphe guttata	Corn snake	North America
Elaphe longissima	Aesculapian snake	Europe, W. Asia, Italy, S. Russia
Elaphe obsoleta	Pilot black snake	North America, Gulf States
Elaphe quadrivittata	Chicken snake	North America
Elaphe quatuorlineata	Aldrovandi's snake	S.E. Europe, W. Asia, S. Russia, Persia
Elaphe radiata (= *Coluber radiatus*)	Rayed snake	S.W. Asia, India, South-West China, Malay States
Elaphe situla	Leopard snake	Southern Europe, West Asia
Elaps (= *Micrurus*)	Coral snakes	Central and South America
Emys orbicularis	Pond tortoise	Europe, W. Asia, North-West Africa
Eretmochelys imbricata	Hawk-billed turtle	Tropical and subtropical seas
Erythrolamprus aesculapii	Red and black coral snake	Tropical America, Brazil, Peru, Guianas
Esox lucius	Pike	Fresh waters, Europe, N. Asia, North America
Eumeces fasciatus	American five-lined skink	Arizona, Canada
	American blue-tailed skink	New England to Florida, Mississippi
Fordonia leucobalia	Fordonia water snake	South Asia, Australasia, Indo-China, Malay States
Fundulus	Tooth carp	Fresh waters, Eastern N. America, West Africa
Gadus aeglefinus	Haddock	Atlantic ocean, North Sea
Gadus morrhua (= *Gadus callarias*)	Atlantic cod	Atlantic ocean
Gasterosteus aculeatus	Three-spined stickleback	Fresh waters, Northern Europe
Gastropyxis smaragdina	Emerald tree snake	Tropical Africa
Gavialis gangeticus	Gharial, Ganges crocodile	Ganges river, India
Gecko gecko (= *Gecko verticillatus*)	Great house gecko	S.E. Asia, N.E. India, Burma, Siam, Malay States
Gehyra multilata (= *Peropus mutilatus*)	Peron's house gecko	Islands of Indian and Pacific ocean, Indo-China, Hawaii, Mexico
Geoemyda trijuga	Ceylon terrapin	South Asia, India, Ceylon, Burma
Gherronotus multicarinatus	Alligator lizard	California
Gherrosaurus	African lizards	Tropical, Southern and South Africa
Glossina palpalis	Tsetse fly	Tropical Africa
Gobio gobio	Gudgeon	Fresh waters, Europe

Zoological names	Trivial names	Main habitat
Goniocephalus	Angle-headed agama	S.E. Asia, East India
Gordius aquaticus	Hair worm, "Water calf"	Fresh waters, temperate zones
Graptemys geographica	Erie map terrapin	North America
Graptemys pseudo-geographica	Small-headed map terrapin	North America
Heloderma suspectum	Gila monster Arizona poisonous lizard	Arizona, Utah, Nevada
Hemichromis bimaculatus	Jewel fish, Red cichlid	River Nile, Sahara rivers, Congo
Hemidactylus frenatus	Bridled house gecko	India,Indo-China,Australia, Malaya, South Africa, Mexico
Heterodon contortrix	Hog-nosed snake, Puffing adder	North America
Heterodon platyrhinos (= *H. contortrix*)	Hog-nosed snake Puffing adder	Southern States of N. America
Hieremys annandalei	Siam turtle	Siam, Cambodia, Malaysia
Hippocampus	Sea horse	Southern European seas
Hippoglossus vulgaris	Halibut	Temperate seas
Homalopsis buccata	Puff-faced water snake	S.E. Asia, Burma to Java, East India
Hydraspis geoffroyana	Geoffroy's terrapin	Southern Brazil
Hydromedusa maximiliani	Maximilian's terrapin	South America, Brazil
Hydromedusa tectifera	Cope's terrapin	Southern Brazil
Hyla arborea	European tree frog	Europe, Temperate Asia, N. Africa
Hyphessobrycon flammeus	Flame or Neon fish	Fresh waters, Brazil
Idus idus (= *Leuciscus idus*)	Ide or Orfe	Fresh waters of Central and N. Europe
Kachuga	Indian terrapin	Northern India, Burma
Katsuwonus pelamis	Skipjack, Bonito	Tropical seas
Kinosternon scorpiodes	Scorpion mud terrapin	South America, Brazil, Guianas
Kinosternon subrubrum	Pennsylvania mud terrapin or Mud turtle	Southern States of North America
Lacerta agilis	Sand lizard	Europe, Asia, Russia
Lacerta muralis	Wall lizard	Europe, S. Russia, Persia, Greece
Lacerta ocellata (= *L. lepida*)	Eyed lizard	Southwestern Europe Northwest Africa
Lacerta viridis	Green lizard	Europe, Asia, Southern Russia, Persia
Lacerta vivipara	Viviparous lizard	Europe, Asia
Lampetra planeri	Brook lamprey	Streams of Europe, Siberia Japan

Zoological names	Trivial names	Main habitat
Lampropeltis calligaster	Red-bellied king snake	North America
Lampropeltis getulus	King snake	North America, Mexico
Latastia longicauda revoili	A lizard	Somaliland
Leiolepisma (= *Lygosoma*)	Slender skink	New Zealand
Lepomis megalotis	Long-eared sunfish	Fresh waters of Eastern N. America
Leptodeira maculata (= *Crotaphopeltis m.*)	Cat's eye snake	South America
Leptopelis aubryi	A tree frog	Cameroon, West Africa
Leuciscus idus (*Idus idus*)	Ide or Orfe	Fresh waters of Central and N. Europe
Leuciscus leuciscus	Dace	Rivers of Central and N. Europe
Leuciscus rutilus (= *Rutilus rutilus*)	Roach	Rivers of North and Central Europe
Lialis jicarii	Jicari's flap-footed lizard	New Guinea
Liolaemus nigromaculatus	Black-spotted lizard	Chile
Liophis andreae	Andrea's Cuban snake	West Indies, Cuba
Liophis anomala	Parana beauty snake	South America, Brazil, Argentine
Liparidae	Snailfishes	Atlantic and Pacific oceans
Liparis vulgaris (= *Liparis liparis*)	Striped sea snailfish	North Atlantic
Lissemys indica	Indian flap-shelled turtle	India, Ceylon, Burma
Lissemys punctata	Asiatic soft-shelled turtle	Pakistan, Indo-China
Lophius piscatorius	Angler fish	European and African marine waters
Loricaria	A catfish	Fresh waters, South America
Lota lota	Burbot	Fresh waters of Europe
Lucioperca lucioperca	Giant pike-perch	Fresh waters of Eastern Europe
Lycodon	Oriental wolf snakes	South Asia, India, Ceylon, Cochin-China, Philippines, Malay States
Lycodon subcinctus	Banded wolf snake	S.E. China, Malay States
Lycognathus cervinus	A snake	Brazil, Bolivia, Guianas, Trinidad
Lygosoma	Slender skink	New Zealand
Lygosoma moco	Moco skink	New Zealand
Lymnaea	Pond snails	Fresh water, Temperate regions
Mabuya agilis	Raddi's skink	Tropical America, Ecuador, Brazil
Mabuya quinquetaeniata	African blue-tailed or five-lined skink	Egypt to Angola, East Africa, Senegambia
Mabuya raddoni	Raddon's skink	West Africa, Sierra Leone, Gabon, Congo
Mabuya striata	Grant's skink or long-toed skink	South and East Africa

Zoological names	Trivial names	Main habitat
Macroclemys temmincki	Alligator snapping turtle	E.North America, Texas, Georgia, Florida, North Missouri
Malaclemys centrata (= *Malacoclemys terrapin*)	Carolina diamond-backed terrapin. Salt-water terrapin	Carolina, Florida
Malapterus electricus	Electric catfish	Tropical Africa
Mastacembelidae	Spiny eels	Fresh waters of India and Africa
Megalobatrachus japonicus (= *M. maximus*)	Giant salamander	Japan
Mehelya capensis	Cape file snake	East Africa, South Africa
Meizodon (= *Natrix*) *longicauda* (= *Natrix fuliginoides*)	Smoky snake	West Africa
Merluccius merluccius	Marine pike, European hake	Atlantic ocean, Mediterranean
Mesoclemmys (= *Hydraspis*) *gibba*	Gordon's terrapin	Brazil, Trinidad, Guianas
Monopeltis	Burrowing lizards	Central Africa
Mugil cephalus	Grey mullet	European, Asiatic and American seas
Mytilus edulis	Common mussel	Lakes and rivers, temperate zone
Naja melanoleuca	Black and white cobra	Tropical Africa
Naja naja	Indian cobra	Southern Asia, India, China, Malaysia
Naja tripudians fasciata	Cobra	India, China
Naja nigricollis	Black-necked cobra	Africa, Egypt, Angola, Transvaal, Natal
Natrix ferox (= *Tropidonotus ferox*)	Fierce snake	West Africa, Sierra Leone, Calabar
Natrix (= *Tropidonotus*) *natrix*	Grass snake	Europe, Central Asia, North East Africa
Natrix olivacea	Black-backed grass snake	Tropical Africa
Natrix piscator	Indian river snake	India, Indo-China, Malay States
Natrix rhombifera	Hallowell's rhomb snake	North America, Mexico
Natrix tigrina	Chinese tiger snake	N.E. Asia, Japan, Korea, China
Natrix vittata	Long-lined snake	Malay States, Java, Celebes
Necturus maculosus	Mudpuppy. Water dog	Southern North America
Nemacheilus barbatula	Stone loach	Fresh waters of Europe
Nematoda	Round worms	Parasitic
Nematomorpha	Gordian worms	Fresh waters, Temperate zones
Notophthalmus meridionalis	Texas newt	Southern States of N. America, Texas
Notopterus	Featherback fish, Razor-finned fish	Fresh waters of India

Zoological names	Trivial names	Main habitat
Ocadia sinensis	Bennet's terrapin	East Asia, China, Formosa
Ophicephalus	Spotted snake-headed fish	Fresh waters of Southern Asia
Ophis merremi	Merrem's Boipeva snake	South America, Brazil
Ophisaurus	Glass snake	Southeastern Europe, S.W. Asia
Osmerus eperlanus	Smelt, Soarling	Coasts of N. and Central Europe
Pelobates fuscus	European spadefoot	Southern Europe, Spain
Pelusios	Box turtles	Africa, N. America
Pelusios (= Sternothaerus) odoratus	Stinkpot, Musk turtle	New England, S. Ontario, S. Florida, Wisconsin, Texas
Pelusios sinuatus	Natal terrapin	S.E. Africa, Natal, Somaliland, Seychelle islands
Pelusios subniger	Black terrapin	West Africa, Liberia, Congo
Perca fluviatilis	Perch	Fresh waters of Europe
Petromyzon marinus	Sea lamprey	Coasts and rivers of Europe and North America
Phelsuma madagascariensis	Green gecko	Seychelles, Madagascar, East coast of Africa
Phoxinus phoxinus	Minnow	Fresh waters of Europe
Phrynosoma coronatum (= Ph. blainvillii)	Blainville's horned lizard	California
Phrynosoma solare	Regal horned lizard	Southern Arizona, N. California, Mexico
Phyllorhynchus	Leafnosed snakes	Southwestern U.S.A.
Physignathus lesueuri	Water dragon	Australia
Pituophis melanoleucus	Northern Pine snake	Southern New Jersey to S. Carolina
Pituophis melanoleucus sayi	Bull snake	U.S.A. Texas to Minnesota
Planorbis	Flat coiled snail	Fresh water of temperate zones
Platemys (= Hydraspis) radiolata	Milkan's terrapin	Brazil
Platydactylus (= Tarentola) mauretanica	Moorish gecko	Mediterranean coast, Spain to Egypt, Dalmatia, Ionian Islands
Pleurodeles waltli	Pleurodele or Spanish newt	Spain, North Africa
Pleuronectes flesus (= Platichthys fl.)	Flounder	European seas and estuaries
Polypterus senegalus	Sail-finned fish	Rivers of tropical West Africa
Proteus anguineus	Olm	Adelsberg cave, Yugoslavia, Carinthia, Dalmatia
Psammodromus algirus	Algerian sand lizard	S.W. Europe, Northwestern Africa
Psammodromus hispanicus	Spanish sand lizard	Iberian peninsula
Psammophis sibilans	Sand snake African beauty snake	Egypt, Senegambia, Angola, Nyasaland

Zoological names	Trivial names	Main habitat
Pseudechis porphyriacus	Purplish death adder	Australia
Pseudemys elegans	Elegant terrapin	North America
Pseudemys floridana	Florida Cooter or Terrapin	Eastern N. America, S. Georgia, Florida
Pseudemys (= Terrapene) ornata	Ornate box turtle or terrapin	Central America, Mexico
Pseudemys scripta elegans	Red-eared turtle	U.S.A. Georgia to North Carolina
Pseudocordylus	Small-scaled girdled lizard "Dasadder"	South Africa, Cape province
Pterophyllum scalare	Angel fish	Fresh waters of Brazil
Ptyas mucosa	Greater Indian Rat snake	Asia, India, Indo-China, Ceylon, Malay States
Putorius putorius (= Mustelus putorius)	Polecat	Europe
Pygosteus pungitius (= Gasterosteus p.)	Ten-spined stickleback	Fresh waters of N. Europe, Baltic sea
Python molurus	Indian python	East India, Ceylon
Python reticulatus	Reticulate python	East India, Burma, Indo-China, Malay States
Python spilotes	Diamond or Carpet python	Australia, New Guinea
Raia erinacea	Little or hedgehog skate	Marine waters, Temperate zones
Rana arvalis (= R. terrestris)	Field frog	Eastern Europe, Western Asia
Rana boyli	Yellow-legged frog	California
Rana catesbeiana	American bull frog	North America
Rana clamitans	Spring frog	North America
Rana dalmatina	Agile frog	Southern Europe
Rana esculenta	Edible frog	Southern Europe
Rana pipiens	Leopard frog	North America
Rana ridibunda	Marsh frog	Eastern Europe, Kent marshes
Rana rugosa	Japanese wart frog	Japan
Rana sylvatica	Eastern wood frog	Canada, U.S.A.
Rana temporaria	Grass frog	Europe, Northern Asia
Rasbora heteromorpha	Harlequin fish Asiatic minnow	Malay peninsula, Sumatra
Rhamphiophis oxyrhynchus	African sharp-snouted snake	Tropical Africa
Rhodeus amarus	Bitterling	Fresh waters of Central Europe
Rutilus rutilus	Roach	Rivers of North and Central Europe
Salamandra atra	Black salamander	Alpine region
Salamandra salamandra (= S. maculosa)	Spotted salamander	Europe
Salmo gairdneri	Rainbow trout	Rivers of North and Western America

Zoological names	Trivial names	Main habitat
Salmo salar	Salmon	Atlantic and rivers of W. Europe and North America
Salmo trutta fario	Common trout, Brown trout	Coast, rivers and streams of Europe and Eastern Asia
Salvelinus fontinalis	Brook trout, Common American char	Rivers and lakes of North America
Sauromalus ater	Chuckawalla lizard	Lower California
Sauromalus varius	Chuckawalla lizard	California
Scaphiophis albopunctata	Beaked snake	East Africa
Scardinius erythrophthalmus	Rudd	Fresh waters of Europe and Asia Minor
Scincus officinalis (= *Scincus scincus*)	Skink	N. Africa, Algeria to Egypt
Sceloporus graciosus	Mountain swift, Graceful fence lizard	Western and Northern U.S.A., California
Sceloporus magister	Desert spiny lizard	Southern States of U.S.A.
Sceloporus spinosus	Spiny fence lizard	Southern States of U.S.A. Mexico
Sceloporus undulatus	Fence lizard	Eastern U.S.A., New Jersey to Florida
Scomber scombrus	Mackerel	Atlantic ocean
Sialis lutaria	Alder fly	Europe
Siebenrockiella crassicollis	Black thick-necked tortoise	Malay peninsula
Silurus glanis	Wels. European catfish	Fresh waters, Central and Eastern Europe
Siredon mexicanum	Axolotl	Mexico
Siren lacertina	Mud eel	Fresh waters of Southern U.S.A.
Sphenodon punctatus	Tuatara lizard	Little islands near New Zealand
Spilotes pullatus	Cainana rat snake	South America
Squalius cephalus (= *Leuciscus cephalus*)	Chub	Rivers of Europe and Asia Minor
Sternotherus carinatus	Keeled-back musk turtle	Southeastern U.S.A.
Sternotherus odoratus	Stink pot, Mud terrapin	Southern States of N. America
Storeria dekayi	De Kay's snake	Northeastern U.S.A., Mexico
Sus scrofa	Wild pig	Europe
Tarentola mauretanica	Moorish gecko	Mediterranean coast, Spain to Egypt, Dalmatia, Ionian islands
Taricha granulosa	Rough-skinned newt	Southeast U.S.A.
Terrapene carolina	Eastern or Carolina box turtle	Eastern States of U.S.A. Maine to Illinois, Tenessee, Georgia
Terrapene major	Gulf coast box turtle Greater American box turtle	Southern States of U.S.A.
Terrapene triunguis	Three-toes box turtle	Southern States of U.S.A.

Zoological names	Trivial names	Main habitat
Testudo denticulata	Brazilian tortoise Hercules tortoise	Tropical America, Guianas, Brazil, N.E. Peru, Venezuela, Colombia, Panama
Testudo elegans	Starred tortoise	India, Ceylon
Testudo elephantina (= *T. gigantea*)	Giant tortoise	Indian ocean islands, Aldabra islands
Testudo elephantopus (= *T. nigrita*)	Porter's blackish tortoise	Galapagos islands, Indefatigable islands
Testudo gigantea (= *T. elephantina*)	Giant tortoise	Indian ocean islands, Aldabra islands
Testudo graeca	Greek tortoise	Southern Europe, North Africa, Western Asia, Near East
Testudo hermanni	Spur-tailed Mediterranean tortoise	Southern Europe, Greece, Albania, Sardinia, Sicily
Testudo marginata	Tafrail tortoise	Southeast Europe, Greece
Thalassochelys caretta (= *Caretta caretta*)	Loggerhead turtle	Tropical and subtropical seas
Thamnophis ordinoides	Elegant garter snake	N.W. America, California
Thamnophis parietalis	Red-sided garter snake	Western North America
Thamnophis radix	Eastern plains garter snake	Eastern North America
Thamnophis sirtalis	Garter snake	North America, Southern Canada, British Columbia
Thymallus thymallus (= *Thymallus vulgaris*)	Grayling	Fresh waters, N. and Central Europe
Tilapia galilea	Galilee cichlid	Northern Israel
Tiliqua scincoides	Northern blue-tongued skink	Australia, Tasmania
Tinca tinca (= *Tinca vulgaris*)	Tench	Fresh waters of Europe, Asia minor and West Siberia
Trachysaurus rugosus	Stump-tailed skink	Australia
Trichogaster leeri	Pearl gourami	Siam, Malaga, Sumatra, Fresh waters
Trichogaster trichopterus	Three-spot gourami	Fresh waters of India, Malaya, Indo-China
Trigla gurnardus	Gurnard	European seas
Trionyx gangeticus	Ganges soft-shelled turtle	India, Ganges water system
Trionyx mutica	Pointed nose soft-shelled turtle	N. America, Mississippi, St. Lawrence
Trionyx sinensis	Chinese soft-shelled turtle	E. Asia, China, Hainan, Formosa, Japan
Trionyx spinifera	Spiny soft-shelled turtle	Mississippi and St. Lawrence basins
Trionyx triunguis	Nile soft-shelled turtle	Tropical Africa
Triturus alpestris	Alpine newt	Central Europe
Triturus cristatus	Crested newt	Europe
Triturus helveticus (= *Tr. palmatus*)	Palmate newt	Europe
Triton taeniatus (= *Triturus vulgaris*)	Common newt	Europe

Zoological names	Trivial names	Main habitat
Triturus vulgaris	Common newt	Europe
Tropidonotus (= *Natrix*) ferox	Fierce snake	West Africa
Tropidonotus (= *Natrix*) natrix	Grass snake	Palaeoarctic regions, Europe, West and Central Asia, Tunisia, Algeria
Tropidurus peruvianus	Lesson's Peruvian lizard	Peru, Chile
Tropidurus torquatus	Wied's ring-necked lizard	Brazil, Guianas
Tupinambis nigropunctatus	Black-pointed Tegu	Guianas, Brazil, Eastern Peru
Tupinambis teguixin	Great Tegu, Teguexin	Uruguay, Brazil, Guianas
Uma notata	Fringe-toed iguana	Southwestern U.S.A.
Unio	Freshwater mussel	Temperate zones, Northern hemisphere
Uromastix acanthinurus	Bell's dabb lizard	Morocco, Algeria
Uromastix hardwicki	General Hardwicke's lizard	Northwest India, Baluchistan
Uta stansburiana	Side-blotched lizard	California
Valvata	Valve snails	Fresh waters, Temperate zones
Vipera aspis	Asp viper	S. Europe, Italy, Balkan States
Vipera aspis hugyi	Asp viper	South Italy, Sicily
Vipera berus	Northern viper or Adder	Europe, Northern Asia
Xantusia henshawi	Henshaw's lizard	Southern California
Xenodon güntheri (= *Ophis g.*)	Günther's snake	South America, Tropical regions
Xenopus laevis	Claw-footed toad. "Platanna"	Cape province
Xiphophorus helleri	Swordtail	Fresh waters, S. Mexico, Guatemala
Zonurus giganteus (= *Cordylus g.*)	Girdled lizard	South Africa

Trivial and Zoological Names

Trivial name	Zoological name
Agama, angle-headed	*Goniocephalus*
Alder fly	*Sialis lutaria*
Axolotl	Larval form of *Ambystoma mexicanum* (= *A. tigrinum*), *Siredon mexicanum*
Cockle, common	*Cardium edule*
Crocodile, estuarine	*Crocodilus porosus*
Crocodile, Ganges	*Gavialis gangeticus*
Crocodile, marsh	*Crocodilus palustris*
Crocodile, Nile	*Crocodilus niloticus*
Eel, blind	*Amphiuma*

Fishes

Angel fish	*Pterophyllum scalare*
Angler	*Lophius piscatorius*
Barbel	*Barbus barbus*
Bitterling	*Rhodeus amarus*
Bleak	*Alburnus alburnus*
Bonito	*Katsuwonus pelamis*
Bowfin	*Amia calva*
Bream	*Abramis brama*
Bream, white	*Blicca björkna*
Burbot	*Lota lota*
Carp	*Cyprinus carpio*
Carp, crucian	*Carassius carassius*
Catfish, European	*Silurus glanis*
Catfish, amphibian	*Clarias.*
Catfish, coat of mail	*Corydoras palaeatus*
Catfish, dwarf	*Ameiurus nebulosus*
Catfish, electric	*Malapterurus electricus*
Chimaera, plow-nosed or Elephant	*Callorhynchus*
Chub	*Squalius cephalus*
Cichlid, Galilee	*Tilapia galilea*
Cod, Atlantic	*Gadus morrhua* (= *G. callarius*)
Conger eel	*Conger conger*
Dace	*Leuciscus leuciscus*
Drum, fresh water, American	*Aplodinotus grunniens*
Eel	*Anguilla anguilla*
Eel, spiny	Mastacembelidae
Featherback	*Notopterus*
Fighting fish, Regan's or Siamese	*Betta splendens*
Flame	*Hyphessobrycon flammeus*
Flounder	*Pleuronectes* (= *Platichthys*) *flesus*
Goldfish	*Carassius carassius*

Trivial name	Zoological name
Fishes—(contd.)	
Gourami, dwarf	*Colisa (= Trichogaster) lalia*
Gourami, pearl	*Trichogaster leeri*
Gourami, three-spot	*Trichogaster (= Osphromenus) tricho-pterus*
Grayling	*Thymallus*
Gudgeon	*Gobio gobio*
Gurnard	*Trigla gurnardus*
Haddock	*Gadus aeglefinus*
Hake, European	*Merluccius merluccius*
Halibut	*Hippoglossus vulgaris*
Harlequin	*Rasbora heteromorpha*
Hatchet belly	*Carnegiella strigata*
Herring	*Clupea harengus*
Ide	*Idus (= Leuciscus) idus*
Jewel fish	*Hemichromis bimaculatus*
Labyrinth fishes	Anabantidae
Lamprey, brook	*Lampetra planeri*
Lamprey, sea	*Petromyzon marinus*
Mackerel	*Scomber scombrus*
Minnow	*Phoxinus phoxinus*
Minnow, Asiatic	*Rasbora heteromorpha*
Mullet, grey	*Mugil cephalus*
Neon fish	*Hyphessobrycon flammeus*
Orfe	*Idus (= Leuciscus) idus*
Perch	*Perca fluviatilis*
Pike	*Esox lucius*
Pike, cichlid	*Crenichla*
Pike, marine	*Merluccius merluccius*
Pike, perch, giant	*Lucioperca lucioperca*
Pope	*Acerina cernua*
Rabbit fish	*Chimaera monstrosa*
Red cichlid	*Hemichromis bimaculatus*
Roach	*Rutilus rutilus (= Leuciscus rutilus)*
Rudd	*Scardinius erythrophthalmus*
Ruffe	*Acerina cernua*
Sail-finned fish	*Polypterus senegalensis*
Salmon	*Salmo salar*
Sea horse	*Hippocampus*
Sea snail, striped	*Liparis vulgaris (= Liparis liparis)*
Sea wolf	*Anarrhichas lùpus*
Skate, little or hedgehog	*Raia erinacea*
Skipjack	*Katsuwonus pelamis*
Smelt or Sparling	*Osmerus eperlanus*
Snail fishes	Liparidae
Spotted, snake-headed fish	*Ophicephalus*
Stickleback, 3-spined	*Gasterosteus aculeatus*
Stickleback, 10-spined	*Pygosteus (= Pungitius) pungitius*
Stone loach	*Nemacheilus barbatula*
Sturgeon	*Acipenser sturio*
Sunfishes	Centrarchidae
Sunfish, long-eared	*Lepomis megalotis*

Trivial name	Zoological name
Fishes—(contd.)	
Swordtail	*Xiphophorus helleri*
Tench	*Tinca tinca* (= *Tinca vulgaris*)
Tooth carps	*Cyprinodontidae*
Top minnow	*Aphanius*
Trout, brook	*Salvelinus fontinalis*
Trout, common	*Salmo trutto fario*
Trout, rainbow	*Salmo gairdneri*
Wels	*Silurus glanis*
Whitefish	*Coregonus vandesius*
Fish louse	*Argulus*
Flatworms	Cestoda (segmented)
Fluke	Trematoda (unsegmented)
Frogs	
Agile	*Rana dalmatica*
Bull, American	*Rana catesbeiana*
Edible	*Rana esculenta*
Field	*Rana arvalis*
Grass	*Rana temporaria*
Leopard	*Rana pipiens*
Marsh	*Rana ridibunda*
Painted	*Discoglossus pictus*
Spadefoot, European	*Pelobates fuscus*
Spring	*Rana clamitans*
Tree, European	*Hyla arborea*
Wart, Japanese	*Rana rugosa*
Wood, Eastern	*Rana sylvatica*
Yellow-legged	*Rana boyli*
Geckos	
Bridled house gecko	*Hemidactylus frenatus*
Great house gecko	*Gecko gecko*
Green gecko	*Phelsuma madagascariensis*
Moorish gecko	*Tarentola mauretanica*
Peron's house gecko	*Gehyra* (= *Peropus*) *mutilatus*
Gharial	*Gavialis gangeticus*
Gila monster	*Heloderma suspectum*
Gordian worms	Nematomorpha
Hair worm	*Gordius aquaticus*
Hardoun	*Agama stellio*
Iguana, desert pygmi	*Dipsosaurus dorsalis*
Iguana, land, Galapagos	*Conolophus subristatus*
Iguana, spiny tailed	*Ctenosaurus acanthura*
Iguanid, fringe-toed	*Uma notata*
Leech, barbel	*Cystobranchus respirans*
Leech, burbot	*Cystobranchus mammillatus*

Trivial name	Zoological name

Lizards

Alligator	*Gherronotus multicarinatus*
Anolis, greater Cuban	*Anolis equestris*
Basilisk, banded	*Basiliscus vittatus*
Black-spotted	*Liolaemus nigromaculatus*
Blainville's horned	*Phrynosoma coronatum*
Burrowing	*Monopeltis*
Chuckawalla	*Sauromalus ater* or *S. varius*
Crag	*Pseudocordylus*
Dabb, Bell's	*Uromastix acanthinurus*
Dasadder	*Pseudocordylus*
Eyed	*Lacerta ocellata* (= *L. lepida*)
Fence	*Sceloporus undulatus*
Flying	*Draco volans*
Galliwasp	*Diploglossus*
General Hardwicke's	*Uromastix hardwicki*
Girdled	*Cordylus* (= *Zonurus*) *giganteus*
Green	*Lacerta viridis*
Henshaw's	*Xanthusia henshawi*
Jicari's flap-footed	*Lialis jicarii*
Lesson's Peruvian	*Tropidurus*
Mountain swift	*Sceloporus graciosus*
Red worm	*Amphisbaena*
Regal, horned	*Phrynosoma solare*
Ring-necked, Wied's	*Tropidurus torquatus*
Sand	*Lacerta agilis*
Sand, Algerian	*Psammodromus algirus*
Sand, Spanish	*Psammodromus hispanicus*
Side-blotched	*Uta stansburiana*
Small-scaled, girdled	*Pseudocordylus*
Spiny, desert	*Sceloporus magister*
Spiny, fence	*Sceloporus spinosus*
Starred	*Agama stellio*
Strand race-runner	*Cnemidophorus lemniscatus*
Surinam	*Ameiva ameiva*
Tuatara	*Sphenodon punctatus*
Viviparous	*Lacerta vivipara*
Wall	*Lacerta muralis*
White, burrowing	*Amphisbaena alba*

Mud eel	*Siren lacertina*
Mudpuppy	*Necturus maculosus*
Mussel, common	*Mytilus edulis*
Mussel, freshwater	*Unio*

Newts

Alpine	*Triturus alpestris*
.Common	*Triturus vulgaris* (= *Tr. taeniatus*)
Crested	*Triturus cristatus*
Japanese	*Cynops pyrrhogaster*
Palmate	*Triturus helveticus* (= *Tr. palmatus*)

Trivial name	Zoological name
Newts—(*contd.*)	
Pleurodele, Spanish	*Pleurodeles waltli*
Red-spotted	*Diemyctilus viridescens*
Rough-skinned	*Taricha granulosa*
Texas	*Notophthalmus meridionalis*
Olm	*Proteus anguineus*
Pheasant, Lady Amherst's	*Chrysolophus amhersti*
Polecat	*Putorius putorius* (= *Mustelus putorius*)
Pig, wild	*Sus scrofa*
Pond snail	*Lymnaea palustris*
Round worms	Nematoda
Salamander	
Black	*Salamandra atra*
Giant	*Megalobatrachus japonicus*
Northern dusky	*Desmognathus fuscus*
Spotted	*Salamandra salamandra* (= *S. maculosa*)
Tiger	*Ambystoma tigrinum*
Skink	
Blue-tailed or five-lined African	*Mabuya quinquetaeniata*
Blue-tailed, American	*Eumeces fasciatus*
Blue-tongued, Northern	*Tiliqua scincoides*
Common	*Scincus officinalis* (= *Sc. scincus*)
Eyed	*Chalcides ocellatus*
Five-lined, American	*Eumeces fasciatus*
Grant's	*Mabuya striata*
Moco	*Lygosoma moco*
Raddi's	*Mabuya agilis*
Raddon's	*Mabuya raddoni*
Slender	*Leiolepisma* (= *Lygosoma*)
Stump-tailed	*Trachysaurus rugosus*
Snail, flat-coiled	*Planorbis*
Snail, valve	*Valvata*
Slow-worm	*Anguis fragilis*
Sow bug	*Asellus aquaticus*
Snakes	
Aesculapian	*Elaphe longissima*
Aldrovandi's	*Elaphe quatuorlineata*
Andrea's Cuban	*Liophis andreae*
Beaked	*Scaphiophis albopunctata*
Beauty, African	*Psammophis sibilans*
Beauty, Parana	*Liophis anomala*
Black, American	*Coluber constrictor*
Black-backed grass	*Natrix olivacea*
Boa constrictor	*Constrictor constrictor*
Bull	*Pituophis melanoleucus*
Chicken	*Elaphe quadrivittata*
Coach, whip	*Coluber flagellum*

Trivial name	Zoological name

Snakes—(contd.)

Cobra, black and white	*Naja melanoleuca*
Cobra, black-necked	*Naja nigricollis*
Black, Indian	*Naja naja* or *Naja tripudians fasciatus*
Corais	*Drymarchon corais*
Coral	*Elaps* (= *Micrurus*)
Coral, red and black	*Erythrolamprus aesculapii*
Corn	*Elaphe guttata*
Cotton-mouthed moccasin	*Agkistrodon piscivorus*
Death adder, purplish	*Pseudechis porphyricus*
de Kaye's	*Storeria dekayi*
Egg-eating	*Dasypeltis scaber*
Emerald tree	*Gastropyxis smaragdina*
Fer-de-lance	*Bothrops atrox* (= *B. jararaca*)
Fierce	*Natrix ferox* (= *Tropidonotus ferox*)
File, Cape	*Mehelya capensis*
Fordonia water	*Fordonia leucobalia*
Garter	*Thamnophis sirtalis*
Garter, Eastern plains	*Thamnophis radix*
Garter, elegant	*Thamnophis ordinoides*
Garter, red-sided	*Thamnophis parietalis*
Glass	*Ophisaurus*
Gopher	*Drymarchon corais*
Grass	*Natrix* (= *Tropidurus*) *natrix*
Green mamba	*Dendraspis angusticeps*
Green, Günther's	*Dipsadoboa unicolor*
Günther's	*Xenodon güntheri*
Hallowell's rhomb	*Natrix rhombifera*
Hog-nosed	*Heterodon contortrix* (= *H. platyrhinus*)
King	*Lampropeltis getulus*
King, red-bellied	*Lampropeltis calligaster*
Leaf-nosed	*Phyllorhynchus*
Leopard	*Elaphe situla*
Lined, African	*Boaedon lineatus*
Long-lined	*Natrix vittata*
Mamba, green	*Dendraspis angusticeps*
Merrem's Boipeva	*Ophis merremi*
Northern pine	*Pituophis melanoleucus*
Pilot-black	*Elaphe obsolita*
Puff adder	*Bitis arietans* (= *Bitis lachesis*)
Puff-faced water	*Homalopsis buccata*
Puffing adder	*Heterodon contortrix* or *H. platyrhinus*
Python, diamond or carpet	*Python spilotes*
Python, Indian	*Python molurus*
Python, reticulate	*Python reticulatus*
Racer	*Coluber constrictor*
Racer, common Malayan	*Elaphe flavolineata*
Rat, Cainana	*Spilotes pullatus*
Rat, greater Indian	*Ptyas mucosus*
Rough-keeled	*Dasypeltis scaber*
Rattlesnake, horned	*Crotalus cerastes*
Rayed	*Coluber radiatus* (= *Elaphe radiata*)

Trivial name	Zoological name

Snakes—(contd.)
  River, Indian — *Natrix piscator*
  Rufescent — *Crotaphopeltis* (= *Leptodeira*) *hotamboeia*
  Sand — *Psammophis sibilans*
  Sharp-snouted, African — *Rhamphiophis oxyrrhynchus*
  Sidewinder — *Crotalus cerastes*
  Sooty — *Boaedon fuliginosus fuliginosus*
  Tiger, Chinese — *Natrix tigrina*
  Water moccasin — *Agkistrodon piscivorus*
  Whip — *Coluber gemonensis*
  Wolf, banded — *Lycodon subcinctus*
  Wolf, oriental — *Lycodon* sp.

Tegu
  Tegu, black-pointed — *Tupinambis nigropunctatus*
  Tegu, great or Teguexin — *Tupinambis teguixin*

Terrapin
  Alligator — *Chelydra serpentina*
  Bennett's — *Ocadia sinensis*
  Black — *Pelusios subniger*
  Caspian — *Clemmys caspica leprosa*
  Ceylon — *Geoemyda trijuga*
  Cope's — *Hydromedusa tectifera*
  Diamond-back, Carolina — *Malaclemys* (= *Malacoclemmys*) *terrapin*
  Elegant — *Pseudemys elegans*
  Erie, map — *Graptemys geographica*
  Florida cooter or terrapin — *Pseudemys floridana*
  Geoffroy's — *Hydraspis geoffroyana*
  Gordon's — *Mesoclemys* (= *Hydraspis*) *gibba*
  Indian — *Kachuga* sp.
  Japanese — *Clemmys japonica*
  Long-necked — *Chelodina longicollis*
  Maximilian's — *Hydromedusa maximiliani*
  Mikan's — *Platemys radiolata*
  Mud, Pennsylvanian — *Kinosternon subrubrum*
  Natal — *Pelusios sinuatus*
  Painted — *Chrysemys picta*
  Scorpion, mud — *Kinosternon scorpioides*
  Small-headed map — *Graptemys pseudogeographica*
  Spanish — *Clemmys leprosa*
  Speckled — *Clemmys guttata*
  Stinkpot, mud — *Sternotherus odoratus*
  Tinamon, banded — *Crypturus noctivagus*

Toad
  American — *Bufo americanus* (= *B. lentiginosus*)
  Claw-footed, S. African — *Xenopus laevis*
  Common African — *Bufo regularis*
  Common, European — *Bufo bufo*
  Fire-belly — *Bombina bombina*

Trivial name	Zoological name

Toads—(*contd.*)
  Giant marine — *Bufo marinus*
  Green — *Bufo viridis*
  Helmet-headed — *Bufo valliceps*
  Indian or common Asiatic — *Bufo melanostictus*
  Midwife — *Alytes obstetricans*
  Mountain — *Bufo boreas*
  Natterjack — *Bufo calamita*
  Northern — *Bufo americanus* (= *B. lentiginosus*)

Tortoises
  Black, thick-necked — *Siebenrockiella crassicollis*
  Brazilian — *Testudo denticulata*
  Giant — *Testudo elephantina* (= *T. gigantea*)
  Greek — *Testudo graeca*
  Hercules — *Testudo denticulata*
  Pond, European — *Emys orbicularis*
  Porter's blackish — *Testudo elephantopus* (= *T. nigrita*)
  Snake — *Chelodina longicollis*
  Spur-tailed mediterranean — *Testudo hermanni*
  Starred — *Testudo elegans*
  Tafrail — *Testudo marginata*

Tsotse fly — *Glossina palpalis*
Tuatara — *Sphenodon punctatus*

Turtles
  Alligator, snapping — *Macroclemys temmincki*
  Box — *Pelusios* sp.
  Box, Carolina — *Terrapene carolina*
  Box, Eastern — *Terrapene carolina*
  Box, Gulf coast — *Terrapene major*
  Box, ornate — *Pseudemys ornata*
  Chinese — *Chinemys reevesii*
  Flap-shelled, Indian — *Lissemys indica*
  Green — *Chelonia mydas* (= *Ch. viridis*)
  Hawk-billed — *Eretmochelys imbricata*
  Keel-back musk — *Sternotherus carinatus*
  Leatherback — *Dermochelys coriacea*
  Loggerhead — *Caretta caretta* (= *Thalassochelys caretta*)
  Mud, Pennsylvanian — *Kinosternon subrubrum*
  Musk — *Pelusios odoratus*
  Red-eared — *Pseudemys scripta elegans*
  Siam — *Hieremys annandalei*
  Snapping — *Chelydra serpentina*
  Soft-shelled, Asiatic — *Lissemys punctata*
  Soft-shelled, Chinese — *Trionyx sinensis*
  Soft-shelled, fierce — *Trionyx* (= *Amyda*) *ferox*
  Soft-shelled, Ganges — *Trionyx gangeticus*
  Soft-shelled, long-headed — *Chitra indica*

Trivial name	Zoological name
Soft-shelled, Nile	*Trionyx triunguis*
Soft-shelled, pointed-nose	*Trionyx mutica*
Soft-shelled, Senegal	*Cyclanorbis senegalensis*
Soft-shelled, spiny	*Trionyx (= Amyda) spinifera*
Stink pot	*Pelusios odoratus*
Three-toed	*Terrapene triunguis*
Vipers	
Asp	*Vipera aspis*
Cape	*Causus rhombeatus*
Carpet	*Echis carinata*
Horned	*Aspis cerastes*
Night (or Night-adder)	*Causus rhombeatus*
Northern (or Adder)	*Vipera berus*
Nose-horned	*Bitis nasicornis*
West African	*Causus lichtensteini*
Water louse	*Asellus aquaticus*
Water calf	*Gordius aquaticus*
Water dog	*Necturus maculatus*
Water dragon	*Physignathus lesueuri*

SUBJECT INDEX